Springer Undergraduate Texts in Mathematics and Technology

More information about this series at http://www.springer.com/series/7438

Timothy G. Feeman

The Mathematics of Medical Imaging

A Beginner's Guide

Second Edition

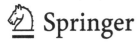 Springer

Timothy G. Feeman
Department of Mathematics and Statistics
Villanova University
Villanova, PA, USA

ISSN 1867-5506   ISSN 1867-5514 (electronic)
Springer Undergraduate Texts in Mathematics and Technology
ISBN 978-3-319-33107-2   ISBN 978-3-319-22665-1 (eBook)
DOI 10.1007/978-3-319-22665-1

Mathematics Subject Classification (2010): 42A38, 42B10, 44A12, 65T50, 68U10, 94A08, 94A20

Springer Cham Heidelberg New York Dordrecht London
© Springer International Publishing Switzerland 2010, 2015
Softcover reprint of the hardcover 2nd edition 2015

Printed on acid-free paper

Springer International Publishing AG Switzerland is part of Springer Science+Business Media (www.springer.
com)

For Max and Simon
and for Alexandra

Contents

Preface to the second edition

In producing this second edition, I acknowledge first and foremost the contributions of the amazing Elizabeth Loew, my editor at Springer. Without her unwavering enthusiasm and support, and, yes, some firm prodding, this project would not have made it this far.

The response I have received to the first edition has been gratifying. I thank the many readers who have sent along their questions, comments, compliments, and lists of typos. All these have been both helpful and encouraging. I have also received repeated requests for any materials I could provide to supplement the text. At first, I had very little available for public consumption. This gradually changed as I used the book myself, for courses at both the undergraduate and master's degree levels. By necessity, I developed additional exercises, created short computer-based assignments, and found new ways to explain some of the tricky concepts. So, in this second edition, I have sought to enhance the development of the main themes and ideas from the earlier edition. This includes the addition of a few new topics that, I hope, lend deeper insight into the core concepts.

Chapter 2 includes new material on the Radon transform and its properties as well as more figures, more worked examples, and a new section that offers a computer-based, hands-on guide to creating phantoms. Chapters 5 and 7 have more on the Dirac delta function and its role in X-ray imaging analysis. Chapter 8 has an expanded look at interpolation using cubic splines, more illustrations of the principal image reconstruction algorithms based on the filtered back projection, and examples of how to implement the algorithms on a computer. Chapter 9, on algebraic image reconstruction techniques, includes more thorough discussions of Kaczmarz's method and least squares approximation, a new section on regularization and spectral filtering, and more computer-based examples and exercises. A new appendix collects some useful results concerning matrices and their transposes that figure in the discussion in Chapter 9, including the eigenvalue decomposition of a (real) symmetric matrix of the form $A^T A$ and the singular value decomposition of a matrix. Additional exercises are to be found in most chapters, with about 30% more exercises overall than in the first edition.

The use of technology has been revamped throughout this second edition, with the incorporation of the open-source programming environment R [42]. I began to study and learn R not too long ago, as part of a research collaboration with a colleague of mine in statistics here at Villanova University. In the midst of running Monte Carlo simulations, I realized that the discrete, vector-based nature of R is well suited to many of the applications found here. Nearly all of the figures have been redesigned using R, and quite a few new figures have been added. More than 20 examples using R are included throughout the text, offering new opportunities for hands-on exploration. SpringerLink includes additional R scripts, including some of those used to produce the figures in the book.

I hope this new edition will stoke your enthusiasm for mathematics and the powerful impact of its applications. Enjoy!

Villanova, PA, USA   Timothy G. Feeman

Preface

In 1979, the Nobel Prize for Medicine and Physiology was awarded jointly to Allan McLeod Cormack and Godfrey Newbold Hounsfield, the two pioneering scientist-engineers primarily responsible for the development, in the 1960s and early 1970s, of computerized axial tomography, popularly known as the CAT or CT scan. In his papers [14], Cormack, then a professor at Tufts University, in Massachusetts, developed certain mathematical algorithms that, he envisioned, could be used to create an image from X-ray data. Working completely independently of Cormack and at about the same time, Hounsfield, a research scientist at EMI Central Research Laboratories in the United Kingdom, designed the first operational CT scanner as well as the first commercially available model. (See [27] and [28].)

Since 1980, the number of CT scans performed each year in the United States has risen from about 3 million to over 67 million. What few people who have had CT scans probably realize is that the fundamental problem behind this procedure is essentially mathematical: If we know the values of the integral of a two- or three-dimensional function along all possible cross sections, then how can we reconstruct the function itself? This particular example of what is known as an *inverse problem* was studied by Johann Radon, an Austrian mathematician, in the early part of the twentieth century. Radon's work incorporated a sophisticated use of the theory of transforms and integral operators and, by expanding the scope of that theory, contributed to the development of the rich and vibrant mathematical field of functional analysis. Cormack essentially rediscovered Radon's ideas, but did so at a time when technological applications were actually conceivable. The practical obstacles to implementing Radon's theories are several. First, Radon's inversion methods assume knowledge of the behavior of the function along every cross section, while, in practice, only a discrete set of cross sections can feasibly be sampled. Thus, it is possible to construct only an approximation of the solution. Second, the computational power needed to process a multitude of discrete measurements and, from them, to obtain a useful approximate solution has been available for just a few decades. The response to these obstacles has been a rich and dynamic development both of theoretical approaches to approximation methods, including the use of interpolation and filters, and of computer algorithms to effectively implement the approximation and inversion strategies. Alongside these mathematical and computational advances, the machines that perform the scans have gone through several generations of improvements in both the speed of data collection and the accuracy of the images, while the range of applications has expanded well beyond the original focus on imaging of the brain. Other related processes, such as positron emission tomography (PET), have developed alongside the advances in CT.

Clearly, this subject crosses many disciplinary boundaries. Indeed, literature on technical aspects of medical imaging appears in journals published in engineering, mathematics, computer science, biomedical research, and physics. This book, which grew out of a course I gave for undergraduate mathematics majors and minors at Villanova University in 2008, addresses the mathematical fundamentals of the topic in a concise way at a relatively elementary level. The emphasis is on the mathematics of CT, though there is also a chapter on magnetic resonance imaging (MRI), another medical imaging process whose originators have earned Nobel prizes. The discussion includes not only the necessary theoretical background but also the role of approximation methods and some attention to the computer implementation of the inversion algorithms. A working knowledge of multivariable calculus and basic vector and matrix methods should serve as adequate prerequisite mathematics.

I hope you will join me, then, in this quest to comprehend one of the most significant and beneficial technological advances of our time and to experience mathematics as an inextricable part of human culture.

Villanova, PA, USA   Timothy G. Feeman

1

X-rays

1.1 Introduction

A computerized axial tomography (CAT or CT) scan is generated from a set of thousands of X-ray beams, consisting of 160 or more beams at each of 180 directions. To comprehend this large collection of X-rays, we must first understand just one beam.

When a single X-ray beam of known intensity passes through a medium, such as muscle or brain tissue or an ancient Egyptian sarcophagus, some of the energy present in the beam is absorbed by the medium and some passes through. The intensity of the beam as it emerges from the medium can be measured by a detector. The difference between the initial and final intensities tells us about the ability of the medium to absorb energy. For the sort of X-rays one might get at the dentist's office or for a suspected broken bone, the detector is a piece of film. A fan- or cone-shaped set of X-rays is emitted from a machine and those photons that are not blocked or absorbed by teeth or bone expose the film, thus creating a picture of the medium. The picture essentially lacks depth since anything positioned behind a point where the photons are blocked will not be seen. This shortcoming highlights a significant difficulty in imaging, namely, that the medium through which the X-rays pass is not homogeneous. For instance, muscles are fibrous and denser in some parts than others; brain tissue is composed of grey matter, water, blood, neurons, and more; inside the sarcophagus is a mummified, partly decomposed body, but also remains of objects that were buried along with the deceased.

The idea behind the CT scan is that, by measuring the changes in the intensity of X-ray beams passing through the medium in different directions and, then, by comparing the measurements, we might be able to determine which locations within the medium are more absorbent or less absorbent than others.

To get an idea of how this works, let's start with a simple model. Suppose we have a one-centimeter-thick slice of material (the medium) in the shape of a square. The square is divided

Electronic supplementary material The online version of this chapter (doi: 10.1007/978-3-319-22665-1_1) contains supplementary material, which is available to authorized users.

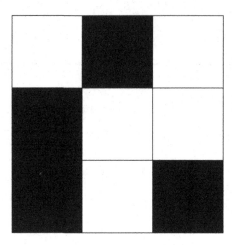

Fig. 1.1. This grid of white and black squares has a prescribed X-ray energy absorption for each row and column.

into a 3-by-3 rectangular grid of smaller squares each of which is either black or white. Each white square absorbs "1 unit" of X-ray energy while the black squares do not absorb X-ray energy. (So the white squares act like bone, say, and the black ones act like air.) Suppose now that an X-ray beam passing through the first row of the grid loses 2 energy units. It follows that there must be two white squares, and one black square, in the first row of the grid. If an X-ray beam passing through the first column of the grid loses 1 unit of energy, then the first column would contain only one white square. At this point, there are only four possibilities for the configuration of the first row and column (instead of the initial $2^5 = 32$ possibilities for these five squares), namely, Row 1 = WWB and Column 1 = WBB; Row 1 = WBW and Column 1 = WBB; Row 1 = BWW and Column 1 = BWB; or Row 1 = BWW and Column 1 = BBW. Continuing in this way, suppose that we measure the following losses in X-ray energy for the various rows and columns of the grid: Row 1 → 2 units lost; Row 2 → 2 units; Row 3 → 1 unit; Column 1 → 1 unit; Column 2 → 2 units; and Column 3 → 2 units of energy lost. Figure 1.1 shows one of several possible configurations of black and white squares that are consistent with these measurements.

What are the other possible configurations? Is there an easy way to determine the total number of white squares, and, consequently, the total number of black squares, in the grid? Is there more than one consistent pattern? If so, what additional information might help to pinpoint a unique shading pattern? For a rich and highly entertaining elaboration on this model for thinking about CT scans, see [16].

In some sense, creating an image from a CT scan consists of carrying out a scheme like this on a rectangular image grid subdivided into thousands of small squares. Instead of just black or white, each square is assigned a greyscale value — a number between 0 and 1, where, by common practice, black is 0 and white is 1 — based on the energy-absorption ability of the material located in that square in the grid. Each X-ray passing through the material is measured, and the change in intensity gives us information about the amount of grey encountered along the path of the beam. What is not known is precisely where along the way the reduction in energy occurred. Once we know the changes in intensity for enough X-rays, we try to create an image whose greyscale values are consistent with the measurements. This approach to image construction is akin to the basic idea implemented by Hounsfield in his early CT scanners and will be discussed in a more refined way in Chapter 9.

Example with R 1.1. There are two ways to produce an image like that in Figure 1.1 using *R*. The `polygon` command allows one to have defined borders within the grid. Otherwise, the `image` command converts a matrix of numbers into a grid of boxes colored according to the matrix entries. The code used here is the following:

```
##Fig 1.1 has three polygonal regions
x1=c(1,0,0,1,1,1,1,2,2,3,3,3,2,2,1)
y1=c(2,2,3,3,2,1,0,0,1,1,2,3,3,2,2)
x2=c(1,0,0,1,1,1,2,2,1)
y2=c(2,2,0,0,2,3,3,2,2)
x3=c(2,2,3,3,2)
y3=c(0,1,1,0,0)
plot(0:3, 0:3, type = "n")
polygon(x1, y1, col = "white",border = "black")
polygon(x2, y2, col = "black",border = "black")
polygon(x3, y3, col = "black",border = "black")
lines(c(1,2,2,3),c(1,1,2,2))
```

1.2 X-ray behavior and Beer's law

To simplify the analysis, we will make some assumptions that present an idealized view of what an X-ray is and how it behaves. Specifically, in thinking of an X-ray beam as being composed of photons, we will assume that the beam is *monochromatic*. That is, each photon has the same energy level E and the beam propagates at a constant frequency, with the same number of photons per second passing through every centimeter of the path of the beam. If $N(x)$ denotes the number of photons per second passing through a point x, then the intensity of the beam at the point x is

$$I(x) = E \cdot N(x).$$

We also assume that an X-ray beam has *zero width* and that it is not subject to refraction or diffraction. That is, X-ray beams are not bent by the medium nor do they spread out as they propagate.

Every substance through which an X-ray passes has the property that each millimeter of the substance absorbs a certain proportion of the photons that pass through it. This proportion, which is specific to the substance, is called the *attenuation coefficient* of that material. The units of the attenuation coefficient are something like "proportion of photons absorbed per millimeter of the medium." In general the attenuation coefficient is non-negative and its value depends on the substance involved. Bone has a very high attenuation coefficient, air has a low

Table 1.1. Approximate Hounsfield units for certain organic substances.

substance	Hounsfield units	substance	Hounsfield units
bone	1000	kidney	30
liver	40 to 60	cerebrospinal fluid	15
white matter	20 to 30	water	0
grey matter	37 to 45	fat	-100 to -50
blood	40	air	-1000
muscle	$10 - 40$		

coefficient, and water is somewhere in between. Different soft tissues have slightly different attenuation coefficients associated with them.

Radiologists actually use a variant of the attenuation coefficient in their work. Developed by Godfrey Hounsfield, the *Hounsfield unit* associated with a medium is a number that represents a comparison of the attenuation coefficient of the medium with that of water. Specifically, the Hounsfield unit of a medium is

$$H_{\text{medium}} := \frac{A_{\text{medium}} - A_{\text{water}}}{A_{\text{water}}}, \tag{1.1}$$

where A denotes the true attenuation coefficient. Table 1.1 gives the Hounsfield units of some typical organic substances.

Now suppose an X-ray beam passes through some medium located between the position x and the position $x + \Delta x$, and suppose that $A(x)$ is the attenuation coefficient of the medium located there. Then the proportion of all photons that will be absorbed in the interval $[x, x + \Delta x]$ is $p(x) = A(x) \cdot \Delta x$. Thus the number of photons that will be absorbed per second by the medium located in the interval $[x, x + \Delta x]$ is $p(x) \cdot N(x) = A(x) \cdot N(x) \cdot \Delta x$. If we multiply both sides by the energy level E of each photon, we see that the corresponding *loss of intensity* of the X-ray beam over this interval is

$$\Delta I \approx -A(x) \cdot I(x) \cdot \Delta x.$$

Let $\Delta x \to 0$ to get the differential equation known as **Beer's law**:

$$\frac{dI}{dx} = -A(x) \cdot I(x) \tag{1.2}$$

This may also be stated as follows.

Beer's law. The rate of change of intensity per millimeter of a nonrefractive, monochromatic, zero-width X-ray beam passing through a medium is jointly proportional to the intensity of the beam and to the attenuation coefficient of the medium. This condition is expressed by the differential equation (1.2).

The differential equation (1.2) is separable and can be written as

$$\frac{dI}{I} = -A(x)\, dx.$$

If the beam starts at location x_0 with initial intensity $I_0 = I(x_0)$ and is detected, after passing through the medium, at the location x_1 with final intensity $I_1 = I(x_1)$, then we get

$$\int_{x_0}^{x_1} \frac{dI}{I} = -\int_{x_0}^{x_1} A(x)\, dx,$$

from which it follows that

$$\ln(I(x_1)) - \ln(I(x_0)) = -\int_{x_0}^{x_1} A(x)\, dx.$$

Thus

$$\ln\left(\frac{I_1}{I_0}\right) = -\int_{x_0}^{x_1} A(x)\, dx.$$

Multiplying both sides by -1 yields the result

$$\int_{x_0}^{x_1} A(x)\, dx = \ln\left(\frac{I_0}{I_1}\right). \tag{1.3}$$

This is a little bit backwards from what we often encounter in textbook problems in differential equations. There, we would typically know the coefficient function and use integration to find the function I. Here, however, we know the initial and final values of I, and it is the coefficient function A, which expresses an essential property of the medium being sampled by the X-ray, that is unknown. Thus, we see that from the measured intensity of the X-ray we are able to determine not the values of A itself, but rather the value of the integral of A along the line of the X-ray.

Example 1.2. For a simple example, suppose the attenuation-coefficient function A is constant throughout a sample. Then, the amount of absorption along any given X-ray beam depends only on the width of the sample along the line of the beam. So, if the beam is travelling along the x-axis and enters the sample at x_0, say, and leaves the sample at x_1, then the amount of absorption is $A(x_1 - x_0)$. It follows from (1.3) that

$$A = \frac{\ln\left(\frac{I_0}{I_1}\right)}{x_1 - x_0},$$

where I_0 and I_1 are the initial and final intensities of the X-ray.

Example 1.3. Suppose that

$$A(x) := \begin{cases} 1 - |x| & \text{if } |x| \leq 1, \\ 0 & \text{if } |x| > 1, \end{cases}$$

and suppose that an X-ray with initial intensity I_0 is emitted at the point x_0 with $x_0 < -1$, passes through the sample, and has final intensity I_1, as measured by a detector at the point x_1 with $x_1 > 1$. Since

$$\int_{x_0}^{x_1} (1 - |x|)\, dx = 1,$$

we see that

$$\ln\left(\frac{I_0}{I_1}\right) = 1,$$

from which it follows that $I_1 = e^{-1} \cdot I_0$. For instance, if $I_0 = 1$, then $I_1 = e^{-1}$. Solving the differential equation $\frac{dI}{dx} = -A(x) \cdot I(x)$, with the initial condition $I_0 = I(-1) = 1$, yields

$$I(x) := \begin{cases} 1 & \text{if } x \leq -1, \\ e^{-x - \frac{1}{2} - \frac{1}{2}x^2} & \text{if } -1 \leq x \leq 0, \\ e^{-x - \frac{1}{2} + \frac{1}{2}x^2} & \text{if } 0 \leq x \leq 1, \\ e^{-1} & \text{if } x \geq 1. \end{cases}$$

Example 1.3: Alternate version. Suppose that the intersection of a sample with the x-axis lies entirely inside the interval $[-1, 1]$ and suppose that an X-ray with initial intensity $I_0 = 1$ is emitted at the point x_0 with $x_0 < -1$, passes through the sample, and has final intensity $I_1 = e^{-1}$, as measured by a detector at the point x_1 with $x_1 > 1$. Moreover, imagine that we somehow knew that the intensity function of the beam was given by

$$I(x) := \begin{cases} 1 & \text{if } x \leq -1, \\ e^{-x - \frac{1}{2} - \frac{1}{2}x^2} & \text{if } -1 \leq x \leq 0, \\ e^{-x - \frac{1}{2} + \frac{1}{2}x^2} & \text{if } 0 \leq x \leq 1, \\ e^{-1} & \text{if } x \geq 1. \end{cases}$$

Beer's law (1.2) now yields

$$A(x) := \begin{cases} 1 - |x| & \text{if } |x| \leq 1, \\ 0 & \text{if } |x| > 1. \end{cases}$$

With actual X-ray detection equipment, though, we would not know the function $I(x)$ at all values of x, only at the points of emission and detection. The condition $I_1 = e^{-1} \cdot I_0$ tells us only that $\int_{x_0}^{x_1} A(x)\, dx = 1$, not what formula $A(x)$ has. For instance, we would not be able to distinguish $A_1(x) := \begin{cases} 1 - |x| & \text{if } |x| \le 1, \\ 0 & \text{if } |x| > 1 \end{cases}$ from $A_2(x) := \begin{cases} 1 & \text{if } |x| \le 1/2, \\ 0 & \text{if } |x| > 1/2 \end{cases}$ or, for that

matter, from any other attenuation function having an integral equal to 1. A single X-ray can measure only the integral of the attenuation function, not its shape.

What we can measure: We can design an X-ray emission/detection machine that can measure the values of I_0 and I_1. Hence, from (1.3), we can compute $\int_{x_0}^{x_1} A(x)\, dx$, the integral of the (unknown) attenuation-coefficient function along the path of the X-ray.

What we want to know: The value of $A(x)$ at each location depends on the nature of the matter located at the point x. It is precisely the function A itself that we wish to know.

Two- or three-dimensional interpretation. Suppose a sample of material occupies a finite region in space. At each point (x, y, z) within the sample, the material there has an attenuation coefficient value $A(x, y, z)$. An X-ray beam passing through the sample follows a line ℓ from an initial point P (assumed to be outside the region) to a final point Q (also assumed to be outside the region). The emission/detection machine measures the initial and final intensities of the beam at P and Q, respectively, from which the value $\ln(I_{\text{initial}}/I_{\text{final}})$ is calculated. According to (1.3), this is equal to the value of the integral $\int_{\overline{PQ}} A(x, y, z)\, ds$, where ds represents arclength units along the segment $\overline{PQ}$ of the line ℓ. Thus, the measurement of each X-ray beam gives us information about the average value of A along the path of the beam.

In our study of CT scans, we will consider a two-dimensional slice of the sample, obtained as the intersection of the sample and some plane, which we will generally assume coincides with the xy-plane. In this context, we interpret the attenuation coefficient function as a function $A(x, y)$ of two variables within the specific slice. Indeed, the word *tomography* is built on the Greek language root form *tomos* meaning "slice."

The fundamental question of image reconstruction is this: *Can we reconstruct the function $A(x, y, z)$ (within some finite region) if we know the average value of A along every line that passes through the region?*

1.3 Lines in the plane

For simplicity, let us assume that we are interested only in the cross section of a sample that lies in the xy-plane. Each X-ray will follow a segment of a line in the plane, so we would like to have a way of cataloguing all such lines. For instance, every nonvertical line has an equation of the form $y = mx + b$. So we could catalogue these lines using all possible pairs (m, b). However, vertical lines would be excluded from this list. Instead, we can classify all lines by adopting a "point–normal" approach, in which every line in the plane is characterized by a pair consisting of a point that the line passes through and a vector that is normal (i.e., perpendicular) to the line.

For a vector $\overrightarrow{n}$ normal to a given line ℓ, there is some angle θ (with $0 \le \theta < 2\pi$, say) such that $\overrightarrow{n}$ is parallel to the line radiating out from the origin at an angle of θ measured

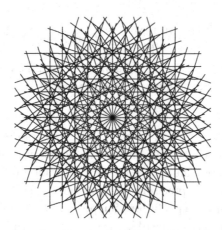

Fig. 1.2. The figure shows the lines $\ell_{t,\theta}$ for eleven different values of t and values of θ in increments of $\pi/10$.

counterclockwise from the positive x-axis. This line, at angle θ, is also perpendicular to ℓ and, hence, intersects ℓ at some point whose coordinates in the xy-plane have the form $(t\cos(\theta), t\sin(\theta))$ for some real number t. In this way, the line ℓ is characterized by the values of t and θ and is accordingly denoted by $\ell_{t,\theta}$. This may also be stated as follows.

Definition 1.4. For any real numbers t and θ, the line $\ell_{t,\theta}$ is the line that passes through the point $(t\cos(\theta), t\sin(\theta))$ and is perpendicular to the unit vector $\overrightarrow{\mathbf{n}} = \langle\cos(\theta), \sin(\theta)\rangle$.

Every line in the plane can be characterized as $\ell_{t,\theta}$ for some values of t and θ.

For example, the line with Cartesian equation $x + y = \sqrt{2}$ is the same as the line $\ell_{1,\pi/4}$. Figure 1.2 shows an array of lines corresponding to eleven different values of t at each of ten angles θ.

Two relationships are apparent, namely,

$$\ell_{t,\theta+2\pi} = \ell_{t,\theta} \text{ and } \ell_{t,\theta+\pi} = \ell_{-t,\theta} \text{ for all } t, \theta.$$

This means that each line in the plane has many different representations of the form $\ell_{t,\theta}$. To avoid this, we can use either of the sets

$$\{\ell_{t,\theta} : t \text{ real}, 0 \le \theta < \pi\} \text{ or } \{\ell_{t,\theta} : t \ge 0, 0 \le \theta < 2\pi\}.$$

For the most part, we will use the former of these sets.

Parameterization of $\ell_{t,\theta}$. To parameterize a line $\ell_{t,\theta}$, observe that the unit vector $\langle-\sin(\theta), \cos(\theta)\rangle$ is perpendicular to the vector $\langle\cos(\theta), \sin(\theta)\rangle$. Thus, every point on $\ell_{t,\theta}$ has the form

$$\langle t\cos(\theta), t\sin(\theta)\rangle + s \cdot \langle-\sin(\theta), \cos(\theta)\rangle$$

for some real number s. That is, the line $\ell_{t,\theta}$ can be parameterized as $(x(s), y(s))$, where $x(s) = t\cos(\theta) - s\sin(\theta)$ and $y(s) = t\sin(\theta) + s\cos(\theta)$ for $-\infty < s < \infty$. Consequently, $\ell_{t,\theta}$ can be described as

$$\ell_{t,\theta} = \{(t\cos(\theta) - s\sin(\theta), \, t\sin(\theta) + s\cos(\theta)) : -\infty < s < \infty\}. \tag{1.4}$$

Note that at every point $(x(s), y(s))$ on $\ell_{t,\theta}$ we get $x^2 + y^2 = t^2 + s^2$.

Example with R 1.5. We can plot a set of lines $\ell_{t,\theta}$ in parameterized form like so.

```
## Figure 1.2: parameterized lines
xray.line=function(t,theta,s){
xval=t*cos(theta)-s*sin(theta)
yval=t*sin(theta)+s*cos(theta)
list(xval=xval,yval=yval) }
######
sval1=(sqrt(2)/200)*(-200:200)#200 pts on each line
thetaval1=(pi/10)*(1:10-1)
tval1=(1/5)*(-5:5)
##plot
plot(c(-1.45,1.45),c(-1.45,1.45),cex=0.,type='n',
    axes=F,asp=1)
for (m in 1:length(tval1)){
for (k in 1:length(thetaval1)){
xray.out=xray.line(tval1[m],thetaval1[k],sval1)
lines(xray.out$xval,xray.out$yval) } }
```

Lines through a fixed point. For an arbitrary point (a, b) in the plane and a given value for θ, there is a unique value of t for which the line $\ell_{t,\theta}$ passes through (a, b). More precisely, there are unique values of both t and s for which

$$a = t\cos(\theta) - s\sin(\theta) \text{ and} \tag{1.5}$$
$$b = t\sin(\theta) + s\cos(\theta).$$

This is a system of two equations in the two unknowns, t and s. The solutions are $t = a\cos(\theta) + b\sin(\theta)$ and $s = -a\sin(\theta) + b\cos(\theta)$. That is, given a, b, and θ,

$$\text{the line } \ell_{a\cos(\theta)+b\sin(\theta),\,\theta} \text{ passes through } (a, b). \tag{1.6}$$

Again, note that $t^2 + s^2 = a^2 + b^2$, a fact that will be used later to implement a change of coordinates from the (x, y) system to the (t, s) framework.

With the parameterization $x(s) = t\cos(\theta) - s\sin(\theta)$ and $y(s) = t\sin(\theta) + s\cos(\theta)$, from (1.4), the arclength element along the line $\ell_{t,\theta}$ is given by

$$\sqrt{\left(\frac{dx}{ds}\right)^2 + \left(\frac{dy}{ds}\right)^2}\, ds = \sqrt{(-\sin(\theta))^2 + (\cos(\theta))^2}\, ds = ds.$$

Therefore, for a given function $A(x, y)$ defined in the plane, we get

$$\int_{\ell_{t,\theta}} A(x,y) = \int_{s=-\infty}^{\infty} A(t\cos(\theta) - s\sin(\theta),\ t\sin(\theta) + s\cos(\theta))\, ds \qquad (1.7)$$

The value of this integral is exactly what an X-ray emission/detection machine measures when an X-ray is emitted along the line $\ell_{t,\theta}$.

We can now rephrase the fundamental question of image reconstruction to ask, "*Can we reconstruct the function $A(x,y)$ (within some finite region of the plane) if we know the value of $\int_{\ell_{t,\theta}} A(x,y)$ for every line $\ell_{t,\theta}$?*"

1.4 Exercises

1. Consider a 3×3 grid in which each of the nine squares is shaded either black or white.

    (a) Find all possible grids for which Rows 1 and 2 each have two white squares and Row 3 has one white square; Column 1 has one white square and Columns 2 and 3 each have two white squares. (Figure 1.1 shows one solution.)

    (b) Find all possible grids for which Rows 1 and 2 each have two white squares and Row 3 has one white square; Columns 1 and 3 each have one white square and Column 2 has three white squares.

2. Find two different 4×4 grids having the same row and column scans; that is, the first row of the first pattern has the same number of white squares as the first row of the second pattern has, and so on.

3. What additional information would help to identify a 3×3 or 4×4 grid uniquely?

4. What does the attenuation coefficient measure?

5. Referring to Table 1.1, why must an image be accurate to within about 10 Hounsfield units in order to be clinically useful?

6. Explain in a few sentences, and with a minimum of mathematical detail, why Beer's law is a plausible model for X-ray attenuation.

7. Let

$$A(x) := \begin{cases} 1 - |x| & \text{if } |x| \le 1, \\ 0 & \text{otherwise} \end{cases}$$

    and

$$I(x) := \begin{cases} 1 & \text{if } x \le -1, \\ e^{-x - \frac{1}{2} - \frac{1}{2}x^2} & \text{if } -1 \le x \le 0, \\ e^{-x - \frac{1}{2} + \frac{1}{2}x^2} & \text{if } 0 \le x \le 1, \\ e^{-1} & \text{if } x \ge 1. \end{cases}$$

(a) Evaluate $\int_{-1}^{1} A(x)\,dx$ and $\ln\left(\frac{I(-1)}{I(1)}\right)$.

(b) Verify that these functions satisfy the differential equation

$$\frac{dI}{dx} = -A(x) \cdot I(x).$$

8. (a) Sketch the graph of the line $\ell_{1/2,\,\pi/6}$. (So $t = 1/2$ and $\theta = \pi/6$ for this line.)

   (b) Determine the y-intercept of the line $\ell_{1/2,\,\pi/6}$.

9. (a) Explain the parameterization

$$\ell_{t,\theta} = \{(t\cos(\theta) - s\sin(\theta),\ t\sin(\theta) + s\cos(\theta)) : -\infty < s < \infty\}.$$

   (b) Prove that $x^2 + y^2 = t^2 + s^2$ at every point (x, y) on $\ell_{t,\theta}$.

10. Find values of t and θ for which the line $\ell_{t,\theta}$ is the same as the line with equation $\sqrt{3}x + y = 4$.

11. Explain why $\ell_{t,\theta} = \ell_{-t,\theta+\pi}$ for all t and all θ. (A sketch might help.)

12. (a) Given a, b, and θ, find t and s so that

$$(a, b) = (t\cos(\theta) - s\sin(\theta),\ t\sin(\theta) + s\cos(\theta)).$$

   That is, solve the system in (1.5) and verify the statement in (1.6).

   (b) Show that $t^2 + s^2 = a^2 + b^2$ for the values you found in part (a).

13. For a fixed value of $R > 0$, let $f(x, y) := \begin{cases} 1 \text{ if } x^2 + y^2 \le R^2, \\ 0 \quad \text{otherwise.} \end{cases}$

   Show that $\int_{\ell_{t,\theta}} f\,ds = \begin{cases} 2\sqrt{R^2 - t^2} & \text{if } |t| \le R, \\ 0 & \text{if } |t| > R. \end{cases}$

14. Discussion: Why does the fundamental question of image reconstruction require that we consider so many lines? Why would a single set of parallel lines not suffice? (Hint: Think about the game we played with the 3-by-3 grid of black and white squares.)

2

The Radon Transform

2.1 Definition

For a given function f defined in the plane, which may represent, for instance, the attenuation-coefficient function in a cross section of a sample, the fundamental question of image reconstruction calls on us to consider the value of the integral of f along a typical line $\ell_{t,\theta}$. For each pair of values of t and θ, we will integrate f along a different line. Thus, we really have a new function on our hands, where the inputs are the values of t and θ and the output is the value of the integral of f along the corresponding line $\ell_{t,\theta}$. But even more is going on than that because we also wish to apply this process to a whole variety of functions f. So really we start by selecting a function f. Then, once f has been selected, we get a corresponding function of t and θ. Schematically,

$$\text{input } f \mapsto \text{output } \left\{ (t, \theta) \mapsto \int_{\ell_{t,\theta}} f \, ds \right\}.$$

This multi-step process is called the *Radon transform*, named for the Austrian mathematician Johann Karl August Radon (1887–1956) who studied its properties. For the input f, we denote by $\mathcal{R}(f)$ the corresponding function of t and θ shown in the schematic. That is, we make the following definition.

Definition 2.1. For a given function f, whose domain is the plane, the Radon transform of f is defined, for each pair of real numbers (t, θ), by

Electronic supplementary material The online version of this chapter (doi: 10.1007/978-3-319-22665-1_2) contains supplementary material, which is available to authorized users.

$$\mathcal{R}f(t,\,\theta) := \int_{\ell_{t,\theta}} f\,ds$$

$$= \int_{s=-\infty}^{\infty} f(t\cos(\theta) - s\sin(\theta),\; t\sin(\theta) + s\cos(\theta))\,ds. \tag{2.1}$$

A few immediate observations are that (i) both f and $\mathcal{R}f$ are functions; (ii) f is a function of the Cartesian coordinates x and y while $\mathcal{R}f$ is a function of the polar coordinates t and θ; (iii) for each choice of f, t, and θ, $\mathcal{R}f(t,\,\theta)$ is a number (the value of a definite integral); (iv) in the integral on the right, the variable of integration is s, while the values of t and θ are preselected and so should be treated as "constants" when evaluating the integral.

We can visualize the Radon transform of a given function by treating θ and t as *rectangular coordinates*. We depict the values of the Radon transform according to their brightness on a continuum of grey values, with the value 0 representing the color *black*, 0.5 representing a neutral grey, and the value 1 representing *white*. Such a graph is called a *sinogram* and essentially depicts all of the data generated by the X-ray emission/detection machine for the given slice of the sample. The choice of the term *sinogram* is no doubt suggested by the symmetry $\mathcal{R}f(-t,\,\theta + \pi) = \mathcal{R}f(t,\,\theta)$ as well as by the appearance of the graphs for some simple examples that we will explore next. Sinograms can also be portrayed in color, using an appropriate segment of the rainbow in place of the grey scale.

2.2 Examples

Example 2.2. As a first example, suppose our patient has a small circular tumor with radius 0.05 centered at the point $(0,\,1)$, and suppose the attenuation-coefficient function f has the constant value 10 there. Now take an arbitrary value of θ. In this case, when $t = \sin(\theta)$, the line $\ell_{t,\theta}$ will pass through $(0,\,1)$ and make a diameter of the circular tumor. Since the diameter of this disc is $2 \cdot (0.05) = 0.1$, we get $\mathcal{R}f(\sin(\theta), \theta) = 10 \cdot (0.1) = 1$. Moreover, for any given θ, the value of $\mathcal{R}f(t,\,\theta)$ will be zero except on the narrow band $\sin(\theta) - 0.05 < t < \sin(\theta) + 0.05$.

Thus, as θ varies from 0 to π, the graph will show a narrow, brighter grey ribbon of width 0.1 centered around $t = \sin(\theta)$. In other words, the graph of $\mathcal{R}f$ in the $(\theta,\,t)$ plane will resemble the graph of the *sine* function. Similarly, the graph in the $(\theta,\,t)$ plane of the Radon transform of a small, bright disc located at $(1,\,0)$ will resemble the graph of the *cosine* function. Figure 2.1 shows the sinograms for these two bright discs. Perhaps these examples helped to motivate the use of the term *sinogram* for the graph of a Radon transform.

In the previous example, we considered an attenuation-coefficient function that had a constant (nonzero) value on a finite region of the plane and the value 0 outside of that region. To attach some terminology to functions of this type, suppose Ω is some finite region in the plane and take f_Ω to be the function that has the value 1 at each point contained in Ω and the

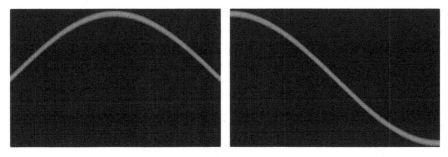

Fig. 2.1. The *sinograms* for small, bright circular discs centered at (0, 1) (left) and at (1, 0) (right) resemble the graphs of the *sine* and *cosine* functions, respectively.

value 0 at each point not in Ω. This function f_Ω is known as the *characteristic function*, or the *indicator function*, of the region Ω. Thus, in our previous example, we looked at 10 times the characteristic function of a small disc.

When the attenuation-coefficient function is a characteristic function f_Ω, its Radon transform is particularly easy to comprehend. Indeed, along any line $\ell_{t,\theta}$, the value of f_Ω will be 0 except when the line is passing through the region Ω, where the value is 1. Thus, for each pair of values of t and θ, the value of $\mathcal{R}f_\Omega(t, \theta)$ *is equal to the length of the intersection of the line $\ell_{t,\theta}$ with the region Ω.*

In general, the object we are testing may comprise a collection of "blobs" of various materials, each with its specific attenuation coefficient. As we shall soon see, the Radon transform of the entire collection will be a composite of the transforms of the separate blobs. Consequently, understanding this basic sort of example will play a central role in assessing the accuracy of various approaches to image reconstruction.

Example 2.3. For instance, let's take the region Ω to be the closed circular disc of radius $R > 0$ centered at the origin. Then the characteristic function of Ω is given by

$$f_\Omega(x, y) := \begin{cases} 1 & \text{if } x^2 + y^2 \leq R^2, \\ 0 & \text{otherwise.} \end{cases}$$

If we choose a value of t such that $|t| > R$, then, regardless of the value of θ, the line $\ell_{t,\theta}$ will not intersect the disc Ω. Thus, $f_\Omega = 0$ at every point on $\ell_{t,\theta}$, and, hence, $\mathcal{R}f_\Omega(t, \theta) = 0$ for such t. On the other hand, if $|t| \leq R$, then $\ell_{t,\theta}$ intersects Ω along the segment corresponding to the parameter values $-\sqrt{R^2 - t^2} \leq s \leq \sqrt{R^2 - t^2}$ in the standard parameterization for the line. The length of this segment is $2\sqrt{R^2 - t^2}$. The value of f_Ω is 1 at points in this interval and 0 otherwise. Therefore, for such t, the value of $\mathcal{R}f_\Omega(t, \theta)$ is the same as the length of the segment, namely, $2\sqrt{R^2 - t^2}$.

In summary, we have shown that

$$\mathcal{R}f_\Omega(t, \theta) = \begin{cases} 2\sqrt{R^2 - t^2} & \text{if } |t| \leq R, \\ 0 & \text{if } |t| > R. \end{cases}$$

Example 2.4. Continuing with the theme of characteristic functions, take S to be the region enclosed by the square whose edges lie along the vertical lines $x = \pm 1$ and the horizontal lines $y = \pm 1$. This square is centered at the origin and has side length 2. Let f_S be the function that takes the value 1 at each point of S and the value 0 at each point not in S. That is, let

$$f_S(x, y) = \begin{cases} 1 & \text{if } \max\{|x|, |y|\} \leq 1, \\ 0 & \text{otherwise.} \end{cases}$$

As discussed above, for each t and each θ, the corresponding value $\mathcal{R}f_S(t, \theta)$, of the Radon transform of f_S, will equal the length of the intersection of the line $\ell_{t,\theta}$ and the square region S. There are two values of θ for which this intersection length is easy to see: $\theta = 0$ and $\theta = \pi/2$. In these cases, the lines $\ell_{t,\theta}$ are vertical or horizontal, respectively. Thus, for $\theta = 0$ or $\theta = \pi/2$, we get $\mathcal{R}f(t, \theta) = 2$ when $-1 \leq t \leq 1$ and $\mathcal{R}f(t, \theta) = 0$ when $|t| > 1$. In general, the function $\mathcal{R}f_S(t, \theta)$ will be piecewise linear in t for each fixed value of θ. Figure 2.2 shows these cross sections for several values of θ.

Figure 2.3 shows the full sinogram for the function f_S. Note the symmetry inherited from that of the square region S. This example will play an important role in the image reconstruction algorithms examined in Chapter 9.

Example 2.5. For an example that is not a characteristic function, let f be the function defined by

$$f(x, y) := \begin{cases} 1 - \sqrt{x^2 + y^2} & \text{if } x^2 + y^2 \leq 1, \\ 0 & \text{if } x^2 + y^2 > 1. \end{cases} \tag{2.2}$$

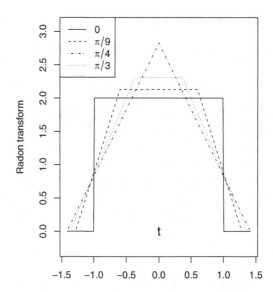

Fig. 2.2. Cross sections at $\theta = 0$, $\theta = \pi/9$, $\theta = \pi/4$, and $\theta = \pi/3$ of the sinogram of the characteristic function of the basic square.

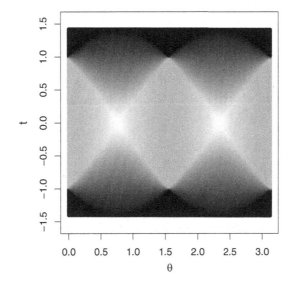

Fig. 2.3. The sinogram for the characteristic function of the square $\mathcal{S} = \{(x, y) : |x| \leq 1, \text{ and } |y| \leq 1\}$.

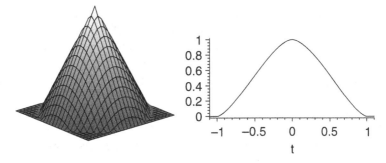

Fig. 2.4. The figure shows the cone defined in (2.2) and the graph of its Radon transform for any fixed value of θ.

The graph of f is a cone, shown in Figure 2.4. We have already observed that, on the line $\ell_{t,\theta}$, we have

$$x^2 + y^2 = (t\cos(\theta) - s\sin(\theta))^2 + (t\sin(\theta) + s\cos(\theta))^2 = t^2 + s^2.$$

It follows that, on the line $\ell_{t,\theta}$, the function f is given by

$$f(t\cos(\theta) - s\sin(\theta),\ t\sin(\theta) + s\cos(\theta))$$

$$:= \begin{cases} 1 - \sqrt{t^2 + s^2} & \text{if } t^2 + s^2 \leq 1, \\ 0 & \text{if } t^2 + s^2 > 1. \end{cases} \tag{2.3}$$

From this, we see that the value of $\mathcal{R}f(t, \theta)$ depends only on t and not on θ and that $\mathcal{R}f(t, \theta) = 0$ whenever $|t| > 1$. For a fixed value of t such that $|t| \leq 1$, the condition $t^2 + s^2 \leq 1$ will be satisfied provided that $s^2 \leq 1 - t^2$. Thus, for any value of θ and for t

such that $|t| \le 1$, we have

$$f(t\cos(\theta) - s\sin(\theta), \ t\sin(\theta) + s\cos(\theta))$$

$$:= \begin{cases} 1 - \sqrt{t^2 + s^2} & \text{if } -\sqrt{1-t^2} \le s \le \sqrt{1-t^2}, \\ 0 & \text{otherwise}; \end{cases} \tag{2.4}$$

whence

$$\int_{\ell_{t,\theta}} f \, ds = \int_{s=-\sqrt{1-t^2}}^{\sqrt{1-t^2}} \left(1 - \sqrt{t^2 + s^2}\right) ds. \tag{2.5}$$

This integral requires a trigonometric substitution for its evaluation. Sparing the details for now, we have

$$\int_{s=-\sqrt{1-t^2}}^{\sqrt{1-t^2}} \left(1 - \sqrt{t^2 + s^2}\right) ds = \sqrt{1-t^2} - \frac{1}{2}t^2 \ln\left(\frac{1 + \sqrt{1-t^2}}{1 - \sqrt{1-t^2}}\right). \tag{2.6}$$

In conclusion, we have shown that the Radon transform of this function f is given by

$$\mathcal{R}f(t, \theta) := \begin{cases} \sqrt{1-t^2} - \frac{1}{2}t^2 \ln\left(\frac{1+\sqrt{1-t^2}}{1-\sqrt{1-t^2}}\right) & \text{if } -1 \le t \le 1, \\ 0 & \text{if } |t| > 1. \end{cases} \tag{2.7}$$

In this case, where $\mathcal{R}f$ is independent of θ, the value of $\mathcal{R}f(t, \theta)$ corresponds to the area under an appropriate vertical cross section of the cone defined by $z = f(x, y)$. Several of these cross sections are visible in Figure 2.4.

2.3 Some properties of $\mathcal{R}$

Suppose that two functions f and g are both defined in the plane. Then so is the function $f + g$. Since the integral of a sum of two functions is equal to the sum of the integrals of the functions separately, it follows that we get, for every choice of t and θ,

$$\mathcal{R}(f + g)(t, \theta) = \int_{s=-\infty}^{\infty} (f + g)(t\cos(\theta) - s\sin(\theta), \ t\sin(\theta) + s\cos(\theta)) \, ds$$

$$= \int_{s=-\infty}^{\infty} \{f(t\cos(\theta) - s\sin(\theta), \ t\sin(\theta) + s\cos(\theta))$$

$$+ g(t\cos(\theta) - s\sin(\theta), \ t\sin(\theta) + s\cos(\theta))\} \, ds$$

$$= \int_{s=-\infty}^{\infty} f(t\cos(\theta) - s\sin(\theta),\ t\sin(\theta) + s\cos(\theta))\, ds$$

$$+ \int_{s=-\infty}^{\infty} g(t\cos(\theta) - s\sin(\theta),\ t\sin(\theta) + s\cos(\theta))\, ds$$

$$= \mathcal{R}f(t,\ \theta) + \mathcal{R}g(t,\ \theta).$$

In other words, $\mathcal{R}(f + g) = \mathcal{R}f + \mathcal{R}g$ as functions.

Similarly, when a function is multiplied by a constant and then integrated, the result is the same as if the function were integrated first and then that value multiplied by the constant; i.e., $\int \alpha f = \alpha \int f$. In the context of the Radon transform, this means that $\mathcal{R}(\alpha f) = \alpha \mathcal{R}f$.

We now have proven the following proposition.

Proposition 2.6. *For two functions f and g and any constants α and β,*

$$\mathcal{R}(\alpha f + \beta g) = \alpha \mathcal{R}f + \beta \mathcal{R}g. \tag{2.8}$$

In the language of linear algebra, we say that the Radon transform is a *linear transformation*; that is, the Radon transform $\mathcal{R}$ maps a linear combination of functions to the same linear combination of the Radon transforms of the functions separately. We also express this property by saying that "$\mathcal{R}$ preserves linear combinations."

Example 2.7. Consider the function

$$f(x,\ y) := \begin{cases} 0.5 & \text{if } x^2 + y^2 \le 0.25, \\ 1.0 & \text{if } 0.25 < x^2 + y^2 \le 1.0, \\ 0 & \text{otherwise.} \end{cases}$$

This a linear combination of the characteristic functions of two circular discs. Namely, $f = f_{\Omega_1} - (0.5)f_{\Omega_2}$, where Ω_1 and Ω_2 are the discs of radii 1 and 0.5, respectively, centered at the origin.

Using property (2.8), along with the computation in Example 2.3, it follows that

$$\mathcal{R}f(t,\ \theta) = \mathcal{R}(f_{\Omega_1})(t,\ \theta) - (0.5)\mathcal{R}(f_{\Omega_2})(t,\ \theta)$$

$$= \begin{cases} 2\sqrt{1-t^2} - \sqrt{(0.25) - t^2} & \text{if } |t| \le 0.5, \\ 2\sqrt{1-t^2} & \text{if } (0.5) < |t| \le 1, \\ 0 & \text{if } |t| > 1. \end{cases}$$

Figure 2.5 shows the graph of this attenuation-coefficient function alongside a graph of the cross section of its Radon transform corresponding to any fixed value of θ and $-1 \le t \le 1$.

What happens to the Radon transform if we modify a function either by shifting it or by re-scaling it? That is, suppose we know the Radon transform of a function f, and now look at the functions $g(x,\ y) = f(x - a,\ y - b)$, where a and b are some real numbers, and $h(x,\ y) = f(cx,\ cy)$, where $c > 0$ is a positive scaling factor.

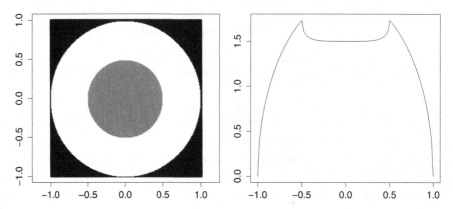

Fig. 2.5. The figure shows the attenuation function defined in Example 2.7 alongside the graph of its Radon transform for any fixed value of θ.

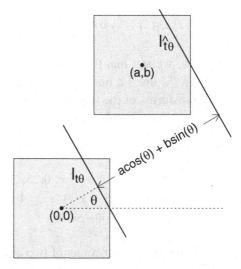

Fig. 2.6. The shifting property of $\mathcal{R}$: The lines $\ell_{t,\theta}$ and $\ell_{t+a\cos(\theta)+b\sin(\theta),\theta}$ intersect congruent regions, centered at $(0, 0)$ and (a, b), respectively, along segments of the same length.

In the first case, we obtain the graph of g by shifting the graph of f by a units in the x direction and b units in the y direction. It follows that if we take any line $\ell_{t,\theta}$ and shift it by just the right amount, we will get a line $\ell_{\hat{t},\theta}$ with the property that $\mathcal{R}g(\hat{t}, \theta) = \mathcal{R}f(t, \theta)$. What is the correct shift in the value of t? Well, when $t = 0$, then $\ell_{0,\theta}$ passes through the origin, while the parallel line $\ell_{a\cos(\theta)+b\sin(\theta),\theta}$ passes through (a, b), as we saw in Exercise 12 of Chapter 1. So, the relationship between $\ell_{0,\theta}$ and the graph of f is the same as that between $\ell_{a\cos(\theta)+b\sin(\theta),\theta}$ and the graph of g. In other words, the correct shift is $\hat{t} = t + a\cos(\theta) + b\sin(\theta)$. Figure 2.6 illustrates this correspondence.

In the case of the function $h(x, y) = f(cx, cy)$, we can think of the domain of h as a $(1/c)$-times scale model of the corresponding domain for f. Thus, to compute the Radon transform of h for a given choice of t and θ, we first have to scale the value of t by the factor c, in order to locate a parallel line that intersects a similar part of the domain of f. Then multiply

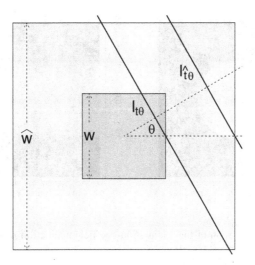

Fig. 2.7. The scaling property of $\mathcal{R}$: With $c = \hat{w}/w = \hat{t}/t$, the length of the intersection of $\ell_{t,\theta}$ with the smaller square region is equal to $1/c$ times the length of the intersection of $\ell_{\hat{t},\theta}$ with the larger square region.

the corresponding value of the Radon transform of f by $1/c$ to get back to the scale of h. That is, for given values of t and θ, we get $\mathcal{R}h(t, \theta) = (1/c) \cdot \mathcal{R}f(ct, \theta)$. This relationship is shown in Figure 2.7, in which f and h are taken to be the characteristic functions of two square regions.

We summarize these statements in a proposition.

Proposition 2.8. *Let the function f be defined in the plane, let a and b be arbitrary real numbers, and let $c > 0$ be a positive real number. Define the function g by $g(x, y) = f(x - a, y - b)$ and the function h by $h(x, y) = f(cx, cy)$. Then, for all real numbers t and θ,*

$$\mathcal{R}g(t, \theta) = \mathcal{R}f(t - a\cos(\theta) - b\sin(\theta), \theta) \text{ and} \tag{2.9}$$

$$\mathcal{R}h(t, \theta) = (1/c) \cdot \mathcal{R}f(ct, \theta). \tag{2.10}$$

Example 2.9. We already know the Radon transform for the characteristic function of a disc of radius $R > 0$ centered at the origin. So now suppose Ω is the disc of radius $R > 0$ centered at (a, b), with characteristic function f_Ω. It follows from (2.9) that the Radon transform of f_Ω is given by

$$\mathcal{R}f_\Omega(t, \theta) = \begin{cases} 2\sqrt{R^2 - \hat{t}^2} & \text{if } |\hat{t}| \leq R, \\ 0 & \text{if } |\hat{t}| > R, \end{cases}$$

where $\hat{t} := t - a\cos(\theta) - b\sin(\theta)$. This certainly looks difficult to compute, but in practice we will use a digital computer, so there is no sweat for us!

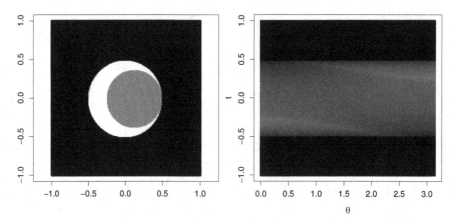

Fig. 2.8. The figure shows the graph of the attenuation-coefficient function A defined in (2.11), alongside a sinogram of its Radon transform $\mathcal{R}A(t, \theta)$.

Example 2.10. To combine several properties of the Radon transform in one example, consider a crescent-shaped region inside the circle $x^2 + y^2 = 1/4$ and outside the circle $(x - 1/8)^2 + y^2 = 9/64$. Assign density 1 to points in the crescent, density $1/2$ to points inside the smaller disc, and density 0 to points outside the larger disc. Thus, the attenuation function is

$$A(x, y) := \begin{cases} 1 & \text{if } x^2 + y^2 \leq 1/4 \text{ and } (x - 1/8)^2 + y^2 > 9/64; \\ 0.5 & \text{if } (x - 1/8)^2 + y^2 \leq 9/64; \\ 0 & \text{if } x^2 + y^2 > 1/4. \end{cases} \qquad (2.11)$$

To break this example into pieces, take Ω_1 to be the closed disc of radius $1/2$ centered at the origin and Ω_2 to be the closed disc of radius $3/8$ centered at $(1/8, 0)$. Then the attenuation function $A(x, y)$ just described can be written as $A(x, y) = f_{\Omega_1}(x, y) - (1/2) \cdot f_{\Omega_2}(x, y)$. It follows from the property (2.8) that, for all t and all θ, $\mathcal{R}A(t, \theta) = \mathcal{R}f_{\Omega_1}(t, \theta) - (1/2) \cdot \mathcal{R}f_{\Omega_2}(t, \theta)$. The second of these two Radon transforms can be computed, as we just discussed, by shifting a Radon transform that we already know, using the property (2.9).

Figure 2.8 shows the graph of this attenuation-coefficient function alongside a graph of its Radon transform in the (t, θ) plane. Figure 2.9 shows graphs of the Radon transform for the angles $\theta = 0$ and $\theta = \pi/3$.

2.4 Phantoms

The fundamental question of image reconstruction asks whether a picture of an attenuation-coefficient function can be generated from the values of the Radon transform of that function. We will see eventually that the answer is *"Yes,"* if all values of the Radon transform are available. In practice, though, only a finite set of values of the Radon transform are measured

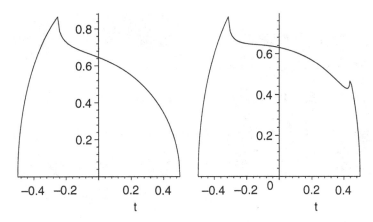

Fig. 2.9. For the function A defined in (2.11), the figure shows graphs of its Radon transform $\mathcal{R}A(t, 0)$ (left) and $\mathcal{R}A(t, \pi/3)$ (right), for $-1/2 \leq t \leq 1/2$.

by a scanning machine, so our answer becomes *"Approximately yes."* Consequently, the nice solution that works in the presence of full information will splinter into a variety of approximation methods that can be implemented when only partial information is at hand.

One method for testing the accuracy of a particular image reconstruction algorithm, or for comparing algorithms, is simply to apply each algorithm to data taken from an actual human subject. The drawback of this approach is that usually we don't know exactly what we ought to see in the reconstructed image. That is what we are trying to find out by creating an image in the first place. But without knowing what the real data are, there is no way to determine the accuracy of any particular image. To get around this, we can apply algorithms to data taken from a physical object whose internal structure is known. That way, we know what the reconstructed image ought to look like and we can recognize inaccuracies in a given algorithm or identify disparities between different algorithms. Nonetheless, this approach can be misleading. Although the internal structure of the object is known, there may be errors in the data that were collected to represent the object. In turn, these errors may lead to errors in the reconstructed image. We will not be able to distinguish these flaws from errors caused by the algorithm itself. To resolve this dilemma, Shepp and Logan, in [49], introduced the concept of a *mathematical phantom*. This is a simulated object, or test subject, whose structure is entirely defined by mathematical formulas. Thus, *no errors occur in collecting the data* from the object. When an algorithm is applied to produce a reconstructed image of the phantom, *all inaccuracies are due to the algorithm.* This makes it possible to compare different algorithms in a meaningful way.

Since measurement of the Radon transform of an object forms the basis for creating a CT image of the object, it makes sense to use phantoms for which the Radon transform is known exactly. We can then test a proposed algorithm by seeing how well it handles the data from such a phantom. For example, we have computed the Radon transform of a circular disc of constant density centered at the origin. Using the linearity of $\mathcal{R}$, along with the shifting and rescaling formulas, we can now compute the Radon transform of any collection of discs, each having constant density, with any centers and radii. More generally,

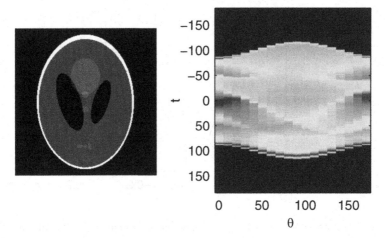

Fig. 2.10. The Shepp–Logan phantom is used as a mathematical facsimile of a brain for testing image reconstruction algorithms. This version of the phantom is stored in MATLAB^R. On the right is a sinogram of the phantom's Radon transform, with θ in increments of $\pi/18$ ($10°$).

the boundary of an arbitrary ellipse is defined by a quadratic expression in x and y. So, as with the circle, determining the intersection of any line $\ell_{t,\theta}$ with an ellipse amounts to finding the difference between two roots of a quadratic equation. In this way, we can calculate exactly the Radon transform of a phantom composed of an assortment of elliptical regions, each having a constant density. Shepp and Logan [49] developed just such a phantom, shown in Figure 2.10.

The Shepp–Logan phantom is composed of eleven ellipses of various sizes, eccentricities, locations, and orientations. (The MATLAB^R version shown here does not include an ellipse that models a blood clot in the lower right near the boundary.) The densities are assigned so that they fall into the ranges typically encountered in a clinical setting. This phantom serves as a useful model of an actual slice of brain tissue and has proven to be a reliable tool for testing reconstruction algorithms.

2.5 Designing phantoms

In this section, we will explore how to design our own phantoms. Each phantom will be a collection of either elliptical regions or square regions, with a constant attenuation-coefficient function on each region. We will find exact formulas for the Radon transforms of these phantoms. This will allow us to plot both the phantom and its sinogram. Indeed, Figures 2.1, 2.3, 2.5, and 2.8 were all created using the templates developed in this section. Like the Shepp–Logan phantom, the phantoms we create here can be used as mathematical models for testing the different image reconstruction algorithms discussed in this book.

2.5.1 *Plotting an elliptical region*

We begin with the problem of designing a phantom made up of elliptical regions. Every ellipse in the xy-plane is determined by the values of five parameters: the lengths a and b of the semi-major and semi-minor axes, the coordinates (x_0, y_0) of the center point of the ellipse, and the angle ϕ of rotation of the axes of the ellipse away from the horizontal and vertical coordinate axes. We can compute coordinates relative to the new center and the rotated framework as

$$\widehat{x} = (x - x_0)\cos(\phi) + (y - y_0)\sin(\phi)\,, \text{ and}$$
$$\widehat{y} = (y - y_0)\cos(\phi) - (x - x_0)\sin(\phi)\,.$$

Then the general formula for the resulting ellipse is given by

$$\frac{\widehat{x}^2}{a^2} + \frac{\widehat{y}^2}{b^2} = 1\,. \tag{2.12}$$

The characteristic function of the region inside the ellipse has value 1 at those points (x, y) for which the expression on the left-hand side of (2.12) is less than or equal to 1, and the value 0 otherwise.

Next, we assign to each region an attenuation-coefficient function that is some constant multiple of the characteristic function for the region. Thus, each elliptical region in the phantom is defined by six values: the five already mentioned along with the attenuation coefficient δ assigned to the region. Our phantom is determined by the sum of the attenuation-coefficient functions of the different regions that make up the phantom. When two regions overlap, the attenuation coefficient on the overlap will be the sum of the individual attenuation coefficients. For instance, we can fashion a skull, as it were, by assigning an attenuation coefficient of 1.0 to a large elliptical region and an attenuation coefficient of, say, -0.9 to a slightly smaller elliptical region inside it. The net effect will be to have a shell with attenuation coefficient 1.0 between the two ellipses (the skull) and a coefficient of $0.1 = 1.0 - 0.9$ inside the shell, where we can place the remaining elements of the phantom.

Example with R 2.11. Figure 2.11 shows a phantom composed of seven elliptical regions each defined by six values $(a, b, x_0, y_0, \phi, \delta)$, as just described. In R, we encode the phantom as a matrix, where each elliptical region defines one row, like so.

```
## each ellipse is a 6-D vector [a,b,x0,y0,phi,greyscale]
p1=c(.7,.8,0,0,0,1)
p2=c(.65,.75,0,0,0,-.9)
p3=c(.15,.2,0,.4,0,.5)
p4=c(.25,.15,-.25,.25,2.37,.2)
p5=c(.25,.15,.25,.25,.79,.2)
p6=c(.08,.25,0,-.3,.5,.65)
p7=c(.05,.05,.5,-.3,0,.8)
#combine into a matrix with one ellipse in each row
P=matrix(c(p1,p2,p3,p4,p5,p6,p7),byrow=T,ncol=6)
```

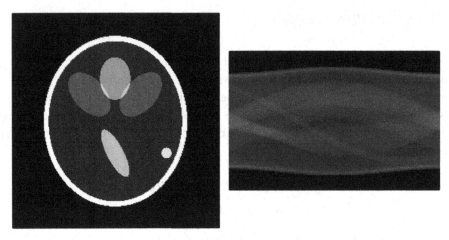

Fig. 2.11. A phantom of elliptical regions; and its sinogram.

Notice the small bright slivers in the top half of the phantom, each formed by the intersection of two of the interior ellipses. These slivers have the attenuation coefficient $0.8 = 0.5 + 0.2 + 1.0 - 0.9$. (Don't forget that both of these ellipses are inside the two ellipses that define the skull.)

To plot the phantom, we need to create a grid of points in the xy-plane that form the locations of the "pixels" in the picture. Here, we first define lists of x and y values in the interval $[-1, 1]$. Then we replicate the full list of x values paired with each y value.

```
##define a K-by-K grid of points in the square [-1,1]x[-1,1]
K=100 #larger K gives better resolution
yval=seq(-1,1,2/K)
grid.y=double((K+1)^2)
for (i in 1:(K+1)^2){
grid.y[i]=yval[floor((i-1)/(K+1))+1]}
xval=seq(-1,1,2/K)
grid.x=rep(xval,K+1)
```

Next, we define a procedure, or function, that checks each point in the grid and adds the attenuation coefficients for those regions that contain it. We apply this function to our phantom to determine the color value for each grid point. Finally, we plot each grid point using a plot character of the assigned color. (The plot character `pch=15` in R is an open square that can be filled with any specified color.)

```
##procedure to compute color value at each grid point
phantom.proc=function(x,y,M){
phantom.1=matrix(double(nrow(M)*length(x)),nrow(M),length(x))
for (i in 1:nrow(M)){
x.new=x-M[i,3]
y.new=y-M[i,4]
phantom.1[i,]=ifelse(M[i,2]^2*(x.new*cos(M[i,5])
+y.new*sin(M[i,5]))^2+M[i,1]^2*(y.new*cos(M[i,5])
```

```
-x.new*sin(M[i,5]))^2-M[i,1]^2*M[i,2]^2<0,M[i,6],0)}
colorvec=colsums(phantom.1)
list(colorvec=colorvec)}#output is "_$colorvec"
# apply the procedure to our phantom P
P.new=phantom.proc(grid.x,grid.y,P)
#create the picture
par(mar=c(0,0,0,0))#removes margins
plot(grid.x,grid.y,pch=15,col=gray(P.new$colorvec))
```

2.5.2 The Radon transform of an ellipse

We now turn our attention to computing the Radon transform of a phantom composed of elliptical regions, each having a constant attenuation coefficient.

To begin with something basic, let $\alpha > 0$ be some positive constant and let $\mathcal{E}_0$ be the closed region bounded by the ellipse with equation $x^2 + \alpha^2 y^2 = \alpha^2$. The characteristic function of $\mathcal{E}_0$ is then

$$f_{\mathcal{E}_0}(x, y) := \begin{cases} 1 & \text{if } x^2 + \alpha^2 y^2 \leq \alpha^2, \\ 0 & \text{otherwise.} \end{cases} \tag{2.13}$$

To determine the Radon transform of $f_{\mathcal{E}_0}$, choose real numbers t and θ, with $0 \leq \theta < \pi$. We give the line $\ell_{t,\theta}$ its usual parameterization:

$$x = t\cos(\theta) - s\sin(\theta); \quad y = t\sin(\theta) + s\cos(\theta); \quad -\infty < s < \infty.$$

Plugging these expressions for x and y into the equation for the boundary ellipse and reorganizing the terms yields a quadratic equation for the parameter s. Specifically, let

$$\begin{aligned} A &= \left(\sin^2(\theta) + \alpha^2 \cos^2(\theta)\right), \\ B &= t\sin(2\theta)\left(\alpha^2 - 1\right), \text{ and} \\ C &= t^2(\cos^2(\theta) + \alpha^2 \sin^2(\theta)) - \alpha^2. \end{aligned} \tag{2.14}$$

Then we wish to find the roots of $A s^2 + B s + C = 0$. (Notice that, if $\alpha = 1$, so that the ellipse is the unit circle, then we get simply $s^2 + t^2 - 1 = 0$, whence, $s = \pm\sqrt{1 - t^2}$. This agrees with our earlier example of a circular region.)

Since $f_{\mathcal{E}_0}$ is the characteristic function of $\mathcal{E}_0$, the value of $\mathcal{R}(f_{\mathcal{E}_0})(t, \theta)$ is equal to the difference between the two roots of this quadratic, in the case where those roots are real numbers, and 0 otherwise. With some persistence, we can express the discriminant of the quadratic as

$$4\alpha^2 \left(\sin^2(\theta) + \alpha^2 \cos^2(\theta) - t^2\right).$$

Thus, we get that

$$\mathcal{R}(f_{\mathcal{E}_0})(t, \theta) = \frac{2\alpha \sqrt{\sin^2(\theta) + \alpha^2 \cos^2(\theta) - t^2}}{\sin^2(\theta) + \alpha^2 \cos^2(\theta)}, \tag{2.15}$$

whenever $t^2 \leq \sin^2(\theta) + \alpha^2 \cos^2(\theta)$, and $\mathcal{R}(f_{\mathcal{E}_0})(t, \theta) = 0$ otherwise. (Again, for $\alpha = 1$, the result is what we got before for the characteristic function of the unit disc.)

Next, consider a more general ellipse, with equation $x^2/a^2 + y^2/b^2 = 1$, and let $\mathcal{E}_1$ be the closed region bounded by this ellipse. Notice that the new region $\mathcal{E}_1$ is a re-scaling by the factor b of the region $\mathcal{E}_0$ bounded by the ellipse $x^2 + \alpha^2 y^2 = \alpha^2$, where $\alpha = a/b$. That is, the point (x, y) lies on the boundary ellipse for $\mathcal{E}_1$ if, and only if, the point $(x/b, y/b)$ lies on the boundary ellipse for $\mathcal{E}_0$. It follows that the characteristic function of the region $\mathcal{E}_1$, denoted by $f_{\mathcal{E}_1}$, satisfies the condition

$$f_{\mathcal{E}_1}(x, y) = f_{\mathcal{E}}(x/b, y/b).$$

Now apply the property (2.10), with $c = 1/b$, to the formula (2.15) above, with $\alpha = a/b$. This gives us the Radon transform of $f_{\mathcal{E}_1}$. Namely,

$$\mathcal{R}(f_{\mathcal{E}_1})(t, \theta) = \frac{2ab \sqrt{b^2 \sin^2(\theta) + a^2 \cos^2(\theta) - t^2}}{b^2 \sin^2(\theta) + a^2 \cos^2(\theta)}, \tag{2.16}$$

whenever $t^2 \leq b^2 \sin^2(\theta) + a^2 \cos^2(\theta)$, and $\mathcal{R}(f_{\mathcal{E}_1})(t, \theta) = 0$ otherwise.

At this point, we have computed the Radon transform of the characteristic function of any ellipse centered at the origin with its major and minor axes lying on the x- and y-coordinate axes. Our next step is to consider an ellipse that is centered at the origin but whose axes lie at an angle from the coordinate axes.

For this, let $\mathcal{E}_1$ denote, as above, the closed region bounded by the ellipse with equation $x^2/a^2 + y^2/b^2 = 1$, and let $\mathcal{E}_\phi$ denote the closed region obtained by rotating $\mathcal{E}_1$ counter-clockwise about the origin by an angle ϕ, with $0 \leq \phi \leq \pi$. It follows that the point (x, y) lies in the region $\mathcal{E}_\phi$ if, and only if, the point $(x\cos(\phi) + y\sin(\phi), -x\sin(\phi) + y\cos(\phi))$ lies in the region $\mathcal{E}_1$. Thus, the characteristic functions of the two regions are related by the equation

$$f_{\mathcal{E}_\phi}(x, y) = f_{\mathcal{E}_1}(x\cos(\phi) + y\sin(\phi), -x\sin(\phi) + y\cos(\phi)).$$

Moreover, for every pair of real numbers t and θ, the intersection of the line $\ell_{t,\theta}$ with the region $\mathcal{E}_\phi$ has the same length as that of the line $\ell_{t,\theta-\phi}$ with the region $\mathcal{E}_1$. Hence, as in Exercise 7 below, we see that

$$\mathcal{R}f_{\mathcal{E}_\phi}(t, \theta) = \mathcal{R}f_{\mathcal{E}_1}(t, \theta - \phi), \text{ for all } t, \theta \in \mathbb{R}.$$

In other words, to compute the Radon transform of $f_{\mathcal{E}_\phi}$, we substitute $\theta - \phi$ for θ in formula (2.16) above.

Finally, we can apply the shifting property (2.9) to obtain the formula for the Radon transform of an elliptical region whose center is located at (x_0, y_0), not necessarily at the origin. In this modification, we replace the value of t by $\hat{t} = t - x_0 \cos(\theta) - y_0 \sin(\theta)$.

To sum up these findings, let $\mathcal{E}$ be the closed region in the xy-plane bounded by the ellipse with center at the point (x_0, y_0) and semi-axes of lengths a and b making an angle of ϕ with the horizontal (x-axis) and vertical (y-axis), respectively. Next, for real numbers t and θ, let $\hat{\theta} = \theta - \phi$ and let $\hat{t} = t - x_0 \cos(\theta) - y_0 \sin(\theta)$. Then, the Radon transform of the characteristic function $f_\mathcal{E}$ is given by

$$\mathcal{R}(f_\mathcal{E})(t, \theta) = \frac{2ab\sqrt{b^2 \sin^2(\hat{\theta}) + a^2 \cos^2(\hat{\theta}) - \hat{t}^2}}{b^2 \sin^2(\hat{\theta}) + a^2 \cos^2(\hat{\theta})}, \tag{2.17}$$

whenever $\hat{t}^2 \le b^2 \sin^2(\hat{\theta}) + a^2 \cos^2(\hat{\theta})$, and $\mathcal{R}(f_\mathcal{E})(t, \theta) = 0$ otherwise. Keep in mind that a computer will evaluate all of this for us!

Remark 2.12. The reader might protest that we could have started with the general formula (2.12) for an ellipse in the plane. After all, computing the Radon transform of the characteristic function of the region inside this ellipse just amounts to finding the distance between two roots of a quadratic equation. This would have led us to the formula (2.17) all at once. This is a fair objection, but it is still fun to solve a simpler quadratic first, and then use the properties of the Radon transform to generalize, isn't it?

Example with R 2.13. Figure 2.11 shows the sinogram of the phantom defined in Example 2.11. The sinogram was produced using R, following a process similar to that used for the image of the phantom itself. This time, we create a grid of values of t and θ corresponding to the lines $\ell_{t,\theta}$ in the "scan" of the phantom, like so.

```
## define values of t and theta for our X-rays
tau=0.02 #space betw/ x-rays
Nangle=180 #no. of angles
Nrays=(1+2/tau)*(Nangle) # total no. of X-rays
tval=seq(-1,1,tau)#for t betw/ -1, 1
thetaval=(pi/Nangle)*(0:(Nangle-1))
## now make a "t, theta" grid:
grid.t=rep(tval,length(thetaval))
grid.theta=double(Nrays)
for (i in 1:Nrays){
grid.theta[i]=thetaval[1+floor((i-1)/length(tval))]}
```

Then we define a procedure that applies formula (2.17) to each elliptical region in the phantom. The results are added together to yield the Radon transform of the full phantom at each point (t, θ). The values of the Radon transform are interpreted as color values in the picture. Finally, we apply this procedure to our particular phantom and plot the resulting sinogram.

```
##this procedure computes the Radon transform
#ellipse parameters stored as rows of matrix E
radon.proc=function(theta,t,E){
tmp=matrix(double(nrow(E)*length(theta)),nrow(E),length
    (theta))
for (i in 1:nrow(E)){
theta.new=theta-E[i,5]
t.new=(t-E[i,3]*cos(theta)-E[i,4]*sin(theta))/E[i,2]
v1=sin(theta.new)^2+(E[i,1]/E[i,2])^2*cos(theta.new)^2-t.
    new^2
v2=ifelse(sin(theta.new)^2
+(E[i,1]/E[i,2])^2*cos(theta.new)^2-t.new^2>0,1,0)
v3=sqrt(v1*v2)
v4=sin(theta.new)^2+(E[i,1]/E[i,2])^2*cos(theta.new)^2
tmp[i,]=E[i,1]*E[i,6]*(v3/v4)}
radvec=colSums(tmp)
list(radvec=radvec)}
##apply the procedure to the phantom P
rp7=radon.proc(grid.theta,grid.t,P)
### plot the sinogram
plot(grid.theta,grid.t,pch=15,col=gray(rp7$radvec))
```

2.5.3 Plotting a square region

We have seen that we can compute the Radon transform of an attenuation-coefficient function that is constant on the region inside an ellipse and zero outside the ellipse. For a region bounded by a polygon, it is a simple matter to determine the point of intersection of any given line $\ell_{t,\theta}$ with each segment of the polygon. By comparing these points, we can determine which segments of $\ell_{t,\theta}$ lie inside the polygonal region. This comparison is easier if the region is convex. Here, we will consider only the example of a square. The attenuation coefficient function under consideration will be a constant multiple of the characteristic function of the region inside the square.

A square in general position in the plane is defined by four parameters: the coordinates (x_0, y_0) of the center of the square, the side length w, and the angle of counterclockwise rotation ϕ from the horizontal. The region inside the square is the set $\{(x, y) \mid \max\{u(x, y), v(x, y)\} < w/2\}$, where

$$u(x, y) = |(x - x_0)\cos(\phi) + (y - y_0)\sin(\phi)| \text{ and}$$

$$v(x, y) = |-(x - x_0)\sin(\phi) + (y - y_0)\cos(\phi)| .$$

This region will be assigned a constant attenuation coefficient, which is interpreted as a color value in the image of the phantom.

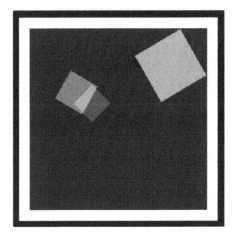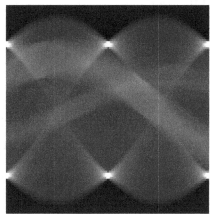

Fig. 2.12. A phantom of square regions; and its sinogram.

Example with *R* 2.14. To create a phantom, we select a set of squares, each determined by five parameters, as just described. In *R*, we can create a matrix in which each row contains the parameters of one square region. As with the ellipses, we examine each point in a grid of "pixels" and add up the attenuation coefficients of all square regions that contain that point. Here is an *R* script that generates the phantom shown in Figure 2.12.

```
##Phantom of squares
##define a grid of points in the square [-1,1]x[-1,1]
K=256 #larger K gives better resolution
yval=seq(-1,1,2/K)
grid.y=double((K+1)^2)
for (i in 1:(K+1)^2){
grid.y[i]=yval[floor((i-1)/(K+1))+1]}
xval=seq(-1,1,2/K)
grid.x=rep(xval,K+1)
##define a phantom using squares, each with 5 parameters
#center (x0, y0);side length w;rotation phi;density
#phantom is a matrix; one row per square
S1=c(0,0,1.9,0,1)
S2=c(0,0,1.7,0,-.9)
S3=c(.5,.5,.5,pi/6,.4)
S4=c(-.25,.15,.25,pi/4,.2)
S5=c(-.4,.25,.3,pi/3,.4)
S=matrix(c(S1,S2,S3,S4,S5),byrow=T,ncol=5)
##check each grid point to see if it is
##inside each square; #add the color values
#use the output "square.out" as the color vector
phantom.square=function(x,y,E){
phantom.1=matrix(double(nrow(E)*length(y)),nrow(E),
```

```
   length(y))
for (i in 1:nrow(E)){
u=abs((x-E[i,1])*cos(E[i,4])+(y-E[i,2])*sin(E[i,4]))
v=abs(-1*(x-E[i,1])*sin(E[i,4])+(y-E[i,2])*cos(E[i,4]))
phantom.1[i,]=E[i,5]*(u<.5*E[i,3])*(v<.5*E[i,3])}
square.out=colSums(phantom.1)
list(square.out=square.out)}
#apply to specific phantom
sq1=phantom.square(grid.x,grid.y,S)$square.out
## plotting the phantom
plot(grid.x,grid.y,pch=20,col=gray(sq1),xlab="",ylab="")
```

2.5.4 The Radon transform of a square region

Now we want to compute the Radon transform of the characteristic function of a square region. As with the ellipses, we'll consider a basic square first. Then we can apply the scaling, shifting, and rotational properties of the Radon transform to solve our problem for a general square.

As in Example 2.4, let S to be the square region whose edges lie along the lines $x = \pm 1$ and $y = \pm 1$, and let f_S denote the characteristic function of S. For each t and each θ, we wish to compute the length of the intersection of the line $\ell_{t,\theta}$ with S. As we observed in Example 2.4,

$$\mathcal{R}f_S(t, 0) = \mathcal{R}f_S(t, \pi/2) = \begin{cases} 2 & \text{if } |t| \leq 1, \\ 0 & \text{if } |t| > 1. \end{cases}$$

More generally, $\mathcal{R}f_S(t, \theta)$ will be piecewise linear in t, as illustrated in Figure 2.2. To generate the sinogram, it is helpful to think of S as the intersection of two infinite bands – the vertical band $V = \{(x, y) : |x| \leq 1\}$ and the horizontal band $H = \{(x, y) : |y| \leq 1\}$. Suppose θ satisfies $0 < \theta < \pi$ and $\theta \neq \pi/2$. In this case, each of the lines $\ell_{t,\theta}$ passes through both of the bands V and H. Indeed, using the standard parameterization of $\ell_{t,\theta}$, we can think of the parameter s as representing time as we travel along the line. Thus, the line crosses the edges of the band V at the times $s_1 = (t \cos(\theta) - 1)/\sin(\theta)$ and $s_2 = (t \cos(\theta) + 1)/\sin(\theta)$. (Note that $\sin(\theta) > 0$ due to our choice of θ.) The lesser of these two time values is the time when $\ell_{t,\theta}$ enters the band V, while the larger time value is the time when $\ell_{t,\theta}$ exits V. Let's denote the entry time by s_{V1} and the exit time by s_{V2}. Similarly, $\ell_{t,\theta}$ crosses the edges of the horizontal band H at the times $s_3 = (-t \sin(\theta) + 1)/\cos(\theta)$ and $s_4 = (-t \sin(\theta) - 1)/\cos(\theta)$. The entry and exit times are given by $s_{H1} = \min\{s_3, s_4\}$ and $s_{H2} = \max\{s_3, s_4\}$, respectively. Now, for the line $\ell_{t,\theta}$ to be inside S, it must be inside both bands V and H simultaneously. For that to happen, both entry times must come before both exit times. (Otherwise, the line would leave one of the bands before it entered the other.) That is, the line $\ell_{t,\theta}$ will intersect the region S if, and only if, $\max\{s_{V1}, s_{H1}\} \leq \min\{s_{V2}, s_{H2}\}$. Then the length of the intersection is just the difference $\min\{s_{V2}, s_{H2}\} - \max\{s_{V1}, s_{H1}\}$. (This is because the standard parameterization is executed at unit speed.) It is straightforward for R to compute these values for each pair (t, θ) included in our CT scan of $\mathcal{S}$. The sinogram for the characteristic function of this basic square is shown in Figure 2.3.

For a square in general position, with center at (x_0, y_0), side length w, and rotation ϕ from the coordinate axes, we calculate entry and exit times as above, but we replace t with $(2/w) \cdot (t - x_0 \cos(\theta) - y_0 \sin(\theta))$ and θ with $\theta - \phi$. (The factor $(2/w)$ is the ratio of the side lengths of the basic square examined above and the new square.) Then we multiply the answer by $(w/2)$, to rescale to our new square. Finally, we multiply by the attenuation coefficient assigned to the region.

Example with R 2.15. To produce the sinogram shown in Figure 2.12, first create a grid of t and θ values, as in Example 2.13. Then we devise a procedure to compute the corresponding values of the Radon transform.

```
##Radon transform for a square region
## assume: values of t and theta are defined
## procedure to compute "entry" and "exit" times
radon.square=function(theta,t,E){
R1=matrix(double(length(theta)*nrow(E)),nrow(E),length
  (theta))
for (i in 1:nrow(E)){
theta.new=theta-E[i,4]
t.new=(t-E[i,1]*cos(theta)-E[i,2]*sin(theta))*(2/E[i,3])
v1=ifelse(theta.new==0,-1*(abs(t.new)<1),
(t.new*cos(theta.new)-1)/sin(theta.new))
v2=ifelse(theta.new==0,1*(abs(t.new)<1),
(t.new*cos(theta.new)+1)/sin(theta.new))
vvmax=ifelse(v1-v2>0,v1,v2)
vvmin=ifelse(v1-v2>0,v2,v1)
h1=ifelse(theta.new==pi/2,-1*(abs(t.new)<1),
(1-t.new*sin(theta.new))/cos(theta.new))
h2=ifelse(theta.new==pi/2,1*(abs(t.new)<1),
-1*(t.new*sin(theta.new)+1)/cos(theta.new))
hhmax=ifelse(h1-h2>0,h1,h2)
hhmin=ifelse(h1-h2>0,h2,h1)
entryval=ifelse(vvmin-hhmin>0,vvmin,hhmin)
exitval=ifelse(vvmax-hhmax>0,hhmax,vvmax)
R1[i,]=(0.5)*E[i,5]*E[i,3]*ifelse(exitval-entryval>0,
(exitval-entryval),0)}
radvec=colSums(R1)
radvec.sq=radvec/max(radvec)#normalizes color vector
list(radvec.sq=radvec.sq)}
## apply radon.square to phantom matrix S
rsq1=radon.square(grid.theta,grid.t,S)
```

```
#plot the sinogram
plot(grid.theta,grid.t,pch=20,
col=gray(rsq1$radvec.sq),xlab=expression(theta),ylab="t")
```

Using the ideas from Examples 2.11, 2.13, 2.14, and 2.15, create some interesting phantoms and sinograms of your own. Use your imagination and have some fun!

2.6 The domain of $\mathcal{R}$

As we can see from the definition (2.1), the Radon transform $\mathcal{R}f$ of a function f is defined provided that the integral of f along $\ell_{t,\theta}$ exists for every pair of values of t and θ. Each of these integrals is ostensibly an improper integral evaluated on an infinite interval. Thus, in general, the function f must be integrable along every such line, as discussed in greater detail in Appendix A.

In the context of medical imaging, the function f represents the density or attenuation-coefficient function of a slice of whatever material is being imaged. Thus, the function has *compact support*, meaning that there is some finite disc outside of which the function has the value 0. In this case, the improper integrals $\int_{\ell_{t,\theta}} f \, ds$ become regular integrals over finite intervals. The only requirement, then, for the existence of $\mathcal{R}f$ is that f be integrable over the finite disc on which it is supported. This will be the case, for instance, if f is piecewise continuous on the disc.

For a wealth of information about the Radon transform and its generalizations, as well as an extensive list of references on this topic, see the monograph [24] and the book [15]. A translation of Radon's original 1917 paper ([43]) into English is included in [15].

2.7 The attenuated Radon transform

The Radon transform is the foundation of our study of computerized tomography when the data we are analyzing come from X-rays that are transmitted externally to the patient or other subject of interest. There are several other forms of tomography, though, in which the data arise from signals that are *emitted from within* the patient. In these so-called *emission tomography* modalities, a radioactive isotope is injected into the patient. The isotope tends to concentrate at sites where a pathology may be present. Thus, we would like to determine the location and distribution of the isotope within the body. Two main variations of emission tomography are *single photon emission computerized tomography*, or SPECT, and *positron emission tomography*, or PET. (A joke: The patient enters the doctor's office and is taken to the examination room. While the patient is waiting, two siamese cats, a schnauzer, and a guinea pig come in, sniff about for a while, and leave. A few moments later, the doctor enters, states that the exam is now concluded, and hands the patient a hefty bill for services rendered. Aghast, the patient exclaims,"But you haven't even examined me!" The doctor replies, "Nonsense! You had both a CAT scan and a PET scan. What more do you want?")

In the case of SPECT, an isotope that emits individual photons, such as iodine–131, is used. When a photon hits the external detector, a device called a *collimator* determines the direction or line of the photon's path. PET uses isotopes that emit positrons, such as carbon–11. Each positron annihilates with a nearby electron to form two γ-rays of known energy and traveling in opposite directions. The simultaneous detection of these γ-rays at opposite detectors determines the line along which the emission took place. In both situations, the count of either photons or γ-rays recorded by each detector corresponds to the measurement of the concentration of the isotope along some portion of the line on which the detector lies. This amounts to knowing the value of the Radon transform along part of that line. The two readings for an opposing pair of positrons combine to give the value of the Radon transform for a full line.

The analysis is complicated by the fact that the medium through which the photons or γ-rays travel, such as the patient's brain perhaps, causes the emitted particles to lose energy. That is, the medium causes attenuation, just as it does for externally transmitted X-rays. The difference is that, with the CT scan based on X-rays, the attenuation coefficient of the medium at each point is the unknown function we wish to find. With emission tomography, it is the unknown location and concentration of the isotope that we wish to determine; but to do that we also have to consider the unknown attenuation coefficient of the medium. To be specific, suppose a photon is emitted at the point (x_0, y_0) and travels along the line $\ell_{t,\theta}$ until it hits the detector. Thus, the photon will pass through all points along $\ell_{t,\theta}$ between (x_0, y_0) and the detector. If (x_0, y_0) corresponds to the parameter value $s = s_0$ in the standard parameterization of $\ell_{t,\theta}$, then the photon will pass through all points of the form $(x, y) = (t\cos(\theta) - s\sin(\theta), t\sin(\theta) + s\cos(\theta))$, for $s \geq s_0$. Denote by $\mu(x, y)$ the attenuation coefficient of the medium at the point (x, y). From Beer's law, it follows that the photon will encounter an attenuation of $\mathcal{A}_\mu(x_0, y_0, t, \theta) = \exp\left[-\int_{s \geq s_0} \mu(x, y)\, ds\right]$, where the integral is evaluated along the portion of $\ell_{t,\theta}$ corresponding to parameter values $s \geq s_0$. Letting $f(x, y)$ denote the (unknown) concentration of radioactive isotope at the point (x, y), we now make the following definition.

Definition 2.16. For a given function f, whose domain is the plane, and a given function μ, the *attenuated Radon transform* of f relative to μ is defined, for each pair of real numbers (t, θ), by

$$\mathcal{R}_\mu f(t, \theta) := \int_{\ell_{t,\theta}} \mathcal{A}_\mu(x, y, t, \theta) f(x, y)\, ds, \tag{2.18}$$

with $\mathcal{A}_\mu$ as just described. If the attenuation of the medium is negligible, so that $\mu(x, y) = 0$, then $\mathcal{A}_\mu = 1$ and $\mathcal{R}_\mu f = \mathcal{R}f$. In general, though, both functions f and μ are unknown. We will not consider these variations on the fundamental question of image reconstruction any further here. More information can be found in the books by Deans [15], Natterer [39], and Kuchment [32].

2.8 Exercises

1. The line $\ell_{1/2,\,\pi/6}$ has the standard parameterization

$$x = \frac{\sqrt{3}}{4} - \frac{s}{2} \text{ and } y = \frac{1}{4} + \frac{\sqrt{3}}{2}s, \text{ for } -\infty < s < \infty.$$

   (a) Find the values of s at which this line intersects the unit circle.

   (b) Now, define f by $f(x,\ y) = \begin{cases} x, & \text{if } x^2 + y^2 \le 1 \\ 0, & \text{if } x^2 + y^2 > 1. \end{cases}$ Compute $Rf(1/2,\ \pi/6)$.

2. Evaluate the integral $\int_{s=-\sqrt{1-t^2}}^{\sqrt{1-t^2}} \left(1 - \sqrt{t^2 + s^2}\right) ds$ from (2.5).

3. As in Example 2.4 above, consider the function

$$f(x,\ y) := \begin{cases} 1 & \text{if } |x| \le 1 \text{ and } |y| \le 1, \\ 0 & \text{otherwise.} \end{cases}$$

   (That is, f has the value 1 inside the square where $-1 \le x \le 1$ and $-1 \le y \le 1$, and the value 0 outside this square.)

   (a) Sketch the graph of the function $Rf(t, 0)$, the Radon transform of f corresponding to the angle $\theta = 0$. Then find a formula for $Rf(t, 0)$ as a function of t.

   (b) Sketch the graph of the function $Rf(t, \pi/4)$, the Radon transform of f corresponding to the angle $\theta = \pi/4$. Then find a formula for $Rf(t, \pi/4)$ as a function of t.

   (c) For θ with $0 \le \theta \le \pi/4$, find relationships, if any, between $Rf(t, \theta)$, $Rf(t, \pi/2-\theta)$, $Rf(t, \theta + \pi/2)$, and $Rf(t, \pi - \theta)$.

4. Show that, for all choices of t and θ and all suitable functions f, $Rf(t, \theta) = Rf(-t, \theta + \pi)$. (This symmetry is one reason that the graph of the Radon transform is called a *sinogram*.)

5. With f as in Example 2.7, find a single disc whose characteristic function g satisfies $Rg(0, \theta) = Rf(0, \theta)$, for all θ. Is $Rg(t, 0) = Rf(t, 0)$ for any values of t with $0 < t < 1$? (*Hint:*Look at the graphs of the Radon transforms.)

6. Provide a rigorous proof of Proposition 2.8 using the definition of the Radon transform as an integral.

7. ($\mathcal{R}$ and rotation.) For a function f defined in the plane and a real number ϕ, define a function g, for all real numbers x and y, by

$$g(x, y) = f(x\cos(\phi) + y\sin(\phi), -x\sin(\phi) + y\cos(\phi)).$$

Thus, the graph of g is a counterclockwise rotation by the angle ϕ of the graph of f. Prove that, for all real numbers t and θ,

$$\mathcal{R}g(t, \theta) = \mathcal{R}f(t, \theta - \phi).$$

3

Back Projection

3.1 Definition and properties

Let us begin the process of trying to recover the values of an attenuation-coefficient function $f(x, y)$ from the values of its Radon transform $\mathcal{R}f$.

Suppose we select some point in the plane, call it (x_0, y_0). This point lies on many different lines in the plane. In fact, for each value of θ, there is *exactly one* real number t for which the line $\ell_{t, \theta}$ passes through (x_0, y_0). Specifically, the value $t = x_0 \cos(\theta) + y_0 \sin(\theta)$ is the one that works, which is to say that, for any given values of x_0, y_0, and θ, the line $\ell_{(x_0 \cos(\theta) + y_0 \sin(\theta)), \theta}$ passes through the point (x_0, y_0). The proof of this fact is left as an exercise.

Example with R 3.1. Figure 3.1 shows a network of back-projection lines through a selection of points in the first quadrant. This figure was created in R with the following code.

```
## plot parameterized lines for the back projection
sval1=(sqrt(2)/100)*(-100:100)#pts on each line
thetaval1=(pi/9)*(1:9-1)#9 angles
#grid of points#plot lines through these
x1=c(rep(0,4),rep(.25,4),rep(.5,4),rep(.75,4))
y1=rep(c(0,.25,.5,.75),4)
plot(c(0,.85),c(0,.85),cex=0.,type='n',xlab='',ylab='',
    asp=1)
for (i in 1:length(x1)){
for (j in 1:Nangle){
xval=(x1[i]*cos(thetaval1[j])+y1[i]*sin(thetaval1[j]))
```

Electronic supplementary material The online version of this chapter (doi: 10.1007/978-3-319-22665-1_3) contains supplementary material, which is available to authorized users.

© Springer International Publishing Switzerland 2015
T.G. Feeman, *The Mathematics of Medical Imaging*, Springer Undergraduate Texts in Mathematics and Technology, DOI 10.1007/978-3-319-22665-1_3

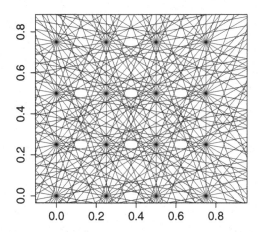

Fig. 3.1. For an array of points in the first quadrant, the figure shows the network of the back-projection lines corresponding to values of θ in increments of $\pi/9$.

```
*cos(thetaval1[j])-sval1*sin(thetaval1[j])
yval=sval1*cos(thetaval1[j])+(x1[i]*cos(thetaval1[j])+y1[i]
*sin(thetaval1[j]))*sin(thetaval1[j])
lines(xval,yval) } }
```

In practice, whatever sort of matter is located at the point (x_0, y_0) in some sample affects the intensity of any X-ray beam that passes through that point. We now see that each such beam follows a line of the form $\ell_{(x_0\cos(\theta)+y_0\sin(\theta)),\theta}$ for some angle θ. In other words, the attenuation coefficient $f(x_0, y_0)$ of whatever is located at the point (x_0, y_0) is accounted for in the value of the Radon transform $\mathcal{R}f(x_0\cos(\theta) + y_0\sin(\theta), \theta)$, for each angle θ.

The first step in recovering $f(x_0, y_0)$ is to compute the *average value* of these line integrals, averaged over all lines that pass through (x_0, y_0). That is, we compute

$$\frac{1}{\pi} \int_{\theta=0}^{\pi} \mathcal{R}f(x_0\cos(\theta) + y_0\sin(\theta), \theta)\, d\theta. \tag{3.1}$$

Formally, this integral provides the motivation for a transform called the back projection, or the back projection transform.

Definition 3.2. Let $h = h(t, \theta)$ be a function whose inputs are polar coordinates. The *back projection* of h at the point (x, y) is defined by

$$\mathcal{B}h(x, y) := \frac{1}{\pi} \int_{\theta=0}^{\pi} h(x\cos(\theta) + y\sin(\theta), \theta)\, d\theta. \tag{3.2}$$

Note that the inputs for $\mathcal{B}h$ are Cartesian coordinates while those of h are polar coordinates.

The proof of the following proposition is left as an exercise.

Proposition 3.3. *The back projection is a linear transformation. That is, for any two functions h_1 and h_2 and arbitrary constants c_1 and c_2,*

$$\mathcal{B}(c_1 h_1 + c_2 h_2)(x, y) = c_1 \mathcal{B} h_1(x, y) + c_2 \mathcal{B} h_2(x, y) \tag{3.3}$$

for all values of x and y.

Example 3.4. Back projection of $\mathcal{R}$. In the context of medical imaging, the integral in (3.1) represents the back projection of the Radon transform of the attenuation-coefficient function f. That is,

$$\mathcal{B}\mathcal{R}f(x, y) = \frac{1}{\pi} \int_{\theta=0}^{\pi} \mathcal{R}f(x \cos(\theta) + y \sin(\theta), \theta) \, d\theta. \tag{3.4}$$

3.2 Examples

Before we rush to the assumption that (3.4) gives us $f(x_0, y_0)$ back again, let us analyze the situation more closely. Each of the numbers $\mathcal{R}f(x_0 \cos(\theta) + y_0 \sin(\theta), \theta)$, themselves the values of integrals, really measures the total accumulation of the attenuation-coefficient function f along a particular line. Hence, the value of the Radon transform along a given line would not change if we were to replace all of the matter there by a homogeneous sample with a constant attenuation coefficient equal to the average of the actual sample's attenuation. The integral in (3.4) now asks us to compute the average value of those averages. Thus, this gives us an "averaged out" or "smoothed out" version of f, rather than f itself. We will make this precise in Proposition 7.20 and its Corollary 7.22. For now, we'll look at some computational examples to illustrate what's going on.

Example 3.5. Suppose f_1 is the attenuation-coefficient function corresponding to a disc of radius $1/2$ centered at the origin and with constant density 1. Then, for every line $\ell_{0,\theta}$ through the origin, we have $\mathcal{R}f_1(0, \theta) = 1$. Consequently, $\mathcal{B}\mathcal{R}f_1(0, 0) = 1$.

Now suppose that f_2 is the attenuation-coefficient function for a ring of width $1/2$ consisting of all points at distances between $1/4$ and $3/4$ from the origin and with constant density 1 in this ring. Then, again, for every line $\ell_{0,\theta}$ through the origin, we get $\mathcal{R}f_2(0, \theta) = 1$. So, again, $\mathcal{B}\mathcal{R}f_2(0, 0) = 1$.

Thus, $\mathcal{B}\mathcal{R}f_1(0, 0) = \mathcal{B}\mathcal{R}f_2(0, 0) = 1$, even though $f_1(0, 0) = 1$ and $f_2(0, 0) = 0$. This illustrates the fact that the back projection of the Radon transform of a function does not necessarily reproduce the original function.

Example 3.6. We previously considered the function

$$f(x, y) := \begin{cases} 1 \text{ if } x^2 + y^2 \leq 1, \\ 0 \quad \text{otherwise} \end{cases}$$

and computed that

$$\mathcal{R}f(t, \theta) = \int_{\ell_{t,\theta}} f \, ds = \begin{cases} 2\sqrt{1 - t^2} & \text{if } |t| \le 1, \\ 0 & \text{if } |t| > 1. \end{cases}$$

From this it follows that, for each point (x, y) and all $0 \le \theta \le \pi$,

$$\mathcal{R}f(x\cos(\theta) + y\sin(\theta), \, \theta)$$
$$= \begin{cases} 2\sqrt{1 - (x\cos(\theta) + y\sin(\theta))^2} & \text{if } |x\cos(\theta) + y\sin(\theta)| \le 1, \\ 0 & \text{if } |x\cos(\theta) + y\sin(\theta)| > 1. \end{cases}$$

It can be pretty difficult to figure out which values of θ satisfy the inequality $|x\cos(\theta) + y\sin(\theta)| \le 1$ for an arbitrary point (x, y). However, the maximum possible value of the expression $|x\cos(\theta) + y\sin(\theta)|$ is $\sqrt{x^2 + y^2}$, and we already know that we only care about points for which $\sqrt{x^2 + y^2} \le 1$. Hence, $|x\cos(\theta) + y\sin(\theta)| \le 1$ will hold for all the points (x, y) that we care about.

Now apply the back projection. Assuming, as we are, that $x^2 + y^2 \le 1$, we get

$$\mathcal{BR}f(x, y) = \frac{1}{\pi} \int_{\theta=0}^{\pi} \mathcal{R}f(x\cos(\theta) + y\sin(\theta), \, \theta) \, d\theta$$
$$= \frac{1}{\pi} \int_{\theta=0}^{\pi} 2\sqrt{1 - (x\cos(\theta) + y\sin(\theta))^2} \, d\theta. \tag{3.5}$$

The three-dimensional graph of f is a circular column of height 1 with a flat top, while the graph of $\mathcal{BR}f$, as Figure 3.2 illustrates, is a circular column with the top rounded off. This is due to the "smoothing" effect of the back projection.

Example 3.7. This time, let

$$f(x, y) := \begin{cases} 1 - \sqrt{x^2 + y^2} & \text{if } x^2 + y^2 \le 1, \\ 0 & \text{otherwise.} \end{cases}$$

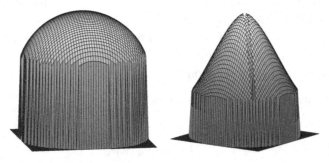

Fig. 3.2. For a test function whose graph is a cylinder or a cone, the back projection of the Radon transform of the function yields a rounded-off cylinder or a rounded-off cone.

In Example 2.5, we computed that, for $-1 \leq t \leq 1$,

$$\mathcal{R}f(t, \theta) = \int_{s=-\infty}^{\infty} f(t\cos(\theta) - s\sin(\theta),\, t\sin(\theta) + s\cos(\theta))\, ds$$

$$= \int_{s=-\sqrt{1-t^2}}^{\sqrt{1-t^2}} \left(1 - \sqrt{t^2 + s^2}\right) ds$$

$$= \sqrt{1 - t^2} - \frac{1}{2}t^2 \ln\left(\frac{1 + \sqrt{1 - t^2}}{1 - \sqrt{1 - t^2}}\right).$$

As in the previous example, the inequality $|x\cos(\theta) + y\sin(\theta)| \leq 1$ is satisfied for all values of θ as long as we only look at points (x, y) in the unit disc. With that assumption, applying the back projection yields

$$\mathcal{B}\mathcal{R}f(x, y) = \frac{1}{\pi} \int_{\theta=0}^{\pi} \mathcal{R}f(x\cos(\theta) + y\sin(\theta),\, \theta)\, d\theta$$

$$= \frac{1}{\pi} \int_{\theta=0}^{\pi} \left\{ \sqrt{1 - t_\theta^2} - \frac{1}{2}t_\theta^2 \ln\left(\frac{1 + \sqrt{1 - t_\theta^2}}{1 - \sqrt{1 - t_\theta^2}}\right) \right\} d\theta,$$

where, for brevity, $t_\theta = x\cos(\theta) + y\sin(\theta)$. If we settle for the use of a Riemann sum, then we can approximate the values of $\mathcal{B}\mathcal{R}f(x, y)$ and generate an approximate graph of $\mathcal{B}\mathcal{R}f(x, y)$ over the unit disc.

In this example, the graph of f is a cone, while the graph of $\mathcal{B}\mathcal{R}f$, shown in Figure 3.2, is a cone that has been rounded off, again illustrating the smoothing effect of the back projection.

In the last two examples above, we restricted the back projection to points (x, y) for which $x^2 + y^2 \leq 1$. For those points, the inequality $|x\cos(\theta) + y\sin(\theta)| \leq 1$ holds for every value of θ. In reality, even for points outside the unit circle, that is, even if $x^2 + y^2 > 1$, there are always *some values* of θ for which $|x\cos(\theta) + y\sin(\theta)| \leq 1$. (For instance, this follows from Exercise 2 below.) For those values of θ, the corresponding line $\ell_{(x\cos(\theta)+y\sin(\theta)),\,\theta}$ passes through the unit disc, and so provides a nonzero value of $\mathcal{R}f(x\cos(\theta) + y\sin(\theta),\, \theta)$. In turn, this nonzero value of the Radon transform contributes to a nonzero value of the back projection $\mathcal{B}\mathcal{R}f(x, y)$. Thus, in the examples above, we have effectively truncated the back projection by "filtering out" points outside the unit circle and excluding them from the smoothing process. The resulting images of $\mathcal{B}\mathcal{R}f$ are actually closer to the original f than if we had not done this filtering. This analysis raises the questions of how we can describe this filtering process mathematically and of whether there are other forms of filtering that will enhance the effort to recover the original attenuation-coefficient function.

Figure 3.3 shows a phantom created in section 2.5. When the back projection is applied to the Radon transform data for the phantom, we see that the bright "skull" in the phantom results in serious distortions. This occurs because every line that intersects the region of the

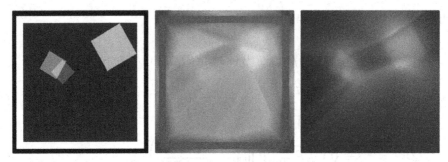

Fig. 3.3. A phantom of squares (left); the back projection of its Radon transform with (center) and without (right) the skull. The presence of the skull interferes with the inversion of the rest of the phantom. Of course, in real life one can't delete the skull!

phantom also intersects the skull. Since the skull is so much brighter than the other features within the phantom, its presence is over-emphasized in the value of the back projection at every point. When the skull is omitted, we get a better reproduction of the phantom, though it is still blurry. (Caution: We can omit the skull only because these are mathematical phantoms. Do not try this on a real human subject!)

Example with R 3.8. The back projection images in Figure 3.3 were formed in R using a discrete form of the back projection that will be discussed in Chapter 8. Essentially, this amounts to replacing the integrals in (3.2) and (3.4) with Riemann sums, taking the angle θ in increments of $d\theta = \pi/N$. We first have to set a grid of points at which to evaluate the back projection, as in Example 2.11. Next, at each point (x, y) in the grid, we compute the average of the values of the integrand at $(x\cos(\theta) + y\sin(\theta), \theta)$ over the various values of θ. Here, the integrand is the Radon transform for the phantom of squares shown in the figure. The following code finishes the process.

```
##Back projection for phantom of squares Fig 3.3
##form K-by-K grid; select theta values:
N=180 # number of angles for the X-rays
theta=pi/N*(1:N-1)
# two matrices: x*cos(theta) and y*sin(theta)
M1=matrix(double((K+1)*N),(K+1),N)
M2=matrix(double((K+1)*N),(K+1),N)
for (i in 1:(K+1)){
M1[i,]=xval[i]*cos(theta)}
for (j in 1:(K+1)){
M2[j,]=yval[j]*sin(theta)}
#phantom of squares; its radon transform
# back projection
bp1=matrix(double((K+1)^2),(K+1),(K+1))
for (i in 1:(K+1)){
for (j in 1:(K+1)){
```

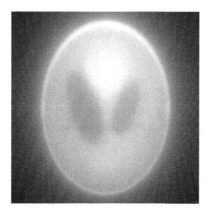

Fig. 3.4. The back projection of the Radon transform of the Shepp–Logan phantom.

```
bp1[i,j]=(1/N)*sum(radon.mat(theta,M1[i,]+M2[j,],S)$radvec
    .sq)}}
# plot the result
plot(grid.x,grid.y,pch=19,cex=1.5,col=gray(bp1),xlab="",
  ylab="")
#re-compute without the skull
```

Example 3.9. The Shepp–Logan phantom. As a final example for now, Figure 3.4 shows the back projection of the Radon transform of the Shepp–Logan phantom, introduced in Figure 2.10. This should reinforce the fact that the back projection is not, by itself, the inverse of the Radon transform. Nonetheless, as we shall see in Chapter 6, the back projection is a crucial ingredient in the image reconstruction process.

3.3 Exercises

1. Verify that, for given values of a, b, and θ, the line $\ell_{(a\cos(\theta)+b\sin(\theta)),\theta}$ passes through the point (a, b).

2. Verify that, for every pair of real numbers a and b, the set of points in the plane that satisfy the polar-coordinate equation

$$r = (a\cos(\theta) + b\sin(\theta)) \text{ for } 0 \leq \theta \leq \pi$$

forms a circle that passes through the origin as well as through the point with Cartesian coordinates (a, b). Find the radius of this circle and the location of its center. (Figure 3.5 illustrates this phenomenon. See [19] for more.)

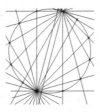

Fig. 3.5. The points where a set of back projection lines intersect their associated radial lines form a circle. See Exercise 2 and [19].

3. (a) For a function $F = F(r, \theta)$, whose inputs are polar coordinates, show that the value of $\mathcal{B}F(x, y)$ is the average value of F on the circle determined by the polar-coordinate equation $r = (x\cos(\theta) + y\sin(\theta))$ for $0 \leq \theta \leq \pi$. (*Hint:* Use Definition 3.2 and Exercise 2.) Use this to compute the following back projections.

   (b) Use part (a) to compute $\mathcal{B}g(x, y)$, where $g(r, \theta) := r\cos(\theta)$.

   (c) Use part (a) to compute $\mathcal{B}h(x, y)$, where $h(r, \theta) := r\sin(\theta)$.

4. Prove Proposition 3.3, which asserts that the back projection is a linear transformation. That is, show that, for any two functions h_1 and h_2 and arbitrary constants c_1 and c_2,

$$\mathcal{B}(c_1 h_1 + c_2 h_2)(x, y) = c_1 \mathcal{B}h_1(x, y) + c_2 \mathcal{B}h_2(x, y)$$

for all values of x and y.

4

Complex Numbers

There is no real number a for which $a^2 + 1 = 0$. In order to develop an expanded number system that includes solutions to this simple quadratic equation, we *define* the "imaginary number" $i = \sqrt{-1}$. That is, this new number i is defined by the condition that $i^2 + 1 = 0$.

Since $i^2 = -1$, it follows that $i^3 = i^2 \cdot i = -1 \cdot i = -i$. Similarly, $i^4 = i^3 \cdot i = -i \cdot i = -i^2 = -(-1) = 1$, and $i^5 = i^4 \cdot i = 1 \cdot i = i$.

As a quick observation, notice that the equation $a^4 = 1$ now has not only the familiar solutions $a = \pm 1$ but also two "imaginary" solutions $a = \pm i$. Thus, there are four *fourth roots of unity*, namely, ± 1 and $\pm i$. The inclusion of the number i in our number system provides us with new solutions to many simple equations.

4.1 The complex number system

The complex number system, denoted by $\mathbb{C}$, is defined to be the set

$$\mathbb{C} = \{a + b \cdot i : a \text{ and } b \text{ are real numbers}\}.$$

To carry out arithmetic operations in $\mathbb{C}$, use the usual rules of commutativity, associativity, and distributivity, along with the definition $i^2 = -1$. Thus, $(a + bi) + (c + di) = (a + c) + (b + d)i$ and $(a + bi) \cdot (c + di) = (ac - bd) + (ad + bc)i$. Also, $-(a + bi) = -a + (-b)i$. Momentarily, we will look at division of one complex number by another.

A geometric view of $\mathbb{C}$. Each complex number $z = a + bi$ is determined by two real numbers. The number a is called the *real part* of z and is denoted by $\Re z = a$, while the number b is called the *imaginary part* and is denoted by $\Im z = b$. (It is important to keep in mind that the imaginary part of a complex number is actually a real number, which is the coefficient of i in the complex number.) In this sense, the complex number system is

© Springer International Publishing Switzerland 2015
T.G. Feeman, *The Mathematics of Medical Imaging*, Springer Undergraduate
Texts in Mathematics and Technology, DOI 10.1007/978-3-319-22665-1_4

"two-dimensional," and so can be represented geometrically in the xy-plane, where we plot the real part of a complex number as the x-coordinate and the imaginary part of the complex number as the y-coordinate.

A real number a can also be written as $a = a + 0 \cdot i$, and so corresponds to the point $(a, 0)$ on the x-axis, which is known therefore as the *real axis*. Similarly, a purely imaginary number $b \cdot i = 0 + b \cdot i$ corresponds to the point $(0, b)$ on the y-axis, which is called the *imaginary axis*.

The distance to the origin from the point (a, b), corresponding to the complex number $a + bi$, is equal to $\sqrt{a^2 + b^2}$. Accordingly, we make the following definition.

Definition 4.1. The *modulus* of the complex number $a + bi$, denoted by $|a + bi|$, is defined by

$$|a + bi| = \sqrt{a^2 + b^2}. \tag{4.1}$$

The modulus of a complex number is analogous to the absolute value of a real number. Indeed, for a real number $a = a + 0 \cdot i$, we get that $|a + 0 \cdot i| = \sqrt{a^2 + 0^2} = |a|$ in the usual sense. Note also that $|a + bi| = 0$ if, and only if, $a = b = 0$. A central observation is that

$$(a + bi) \cdot (a - bi) = a^2 + b^2 = |a + bi|^2.$$

With this in mind, we make another definition.

Definition 4.2. The *conjugate* of a complex number $a + bi$, denoted by $\overline{a + bi}$, is defined by

$$\overline{a + bi} = a - bi. \tag{4.2}$$

The central property, to repeat, is that

$$(a + bi) \cdot \overline{(a + bi)} = (a + bi) \cdot (a - bi) = a^2 + b^2 = |a + bi|^2. \tag{4.3}$$

The conjugate of a complex number is the key ingredient when it comes to the arithmetic operation of division. For example, notice that

$$(5 + 12i)(5 - 12i) = 5^2 + 12^2 = 13^2 = 169.$$

It follows from this that

$$\frac{1}{5 + 12i} = \frac{5 - 12i}{169} = \frac{5}{169} - \frac{12}{169}i,$$

whence

$$\frac{3 + 4i}{5 + 12i} = (3 + 4i) \cdot \frac{1}{5 + 12i} = (3 + 4i)\left(\frac{5}{169} - \frac{12}{169}i\right) = \frac{63}{169} - \frac{16}{169}i.$$

In general, we get that

$$\frac{1}{a+bi} = \frac{1}{a^2+b^2}(a-bi).$$

This enables us to divide any complex number by $(a+bi)$, provided that a and b are not both 0. The act of dividing by the nonzero complex number $(a+bi)$ is re-expressed as multiplication by $(a-bi)$ and division by the nonzero real number (a^2+b^2).

4.2 The complex exponential function

Consider these well-known Taylor series:

$$\cos(x) = \sum_{n=0}^{\infty}(-1)^n\frac{x^{2n}}{(2n)!} = 1 - \frac{x^2}{2!} + \frac{x^4}{4!} - \frac{x^6}{6!} + \cdots,$$

$$\sin(x) = \sum_{n=0}^{\infty}(-1)^n\frac{x^{2n+1}}{(2n+1)!} = x - \frac{x^3}{3!} + \frac{x^5}{5!} - \frac{x^7}{7!} + \cdots,$$

and

$$\exp(x) = e^x = \sum_{n=0}^{\infty}\frac{x^n}{n!} = 1 + x + \frac{x^2}{2!} + \frac{x^3}{3!} + \frac{x^4}{4!} + \cdots.$$

Substitute $x = i\theta$ (where θ is assumed to be a real number) into the series for $\exp(x)$ to get (formally)

$$\exp(i\theta) = e^{i\theta} = \sum_{n=0}^{\infty}\frac{(i\theta)^n}{n!}$$

$$= 1 + (i\theta) + \frac{(i\theta)^2}{2!} + \frac{(i\theta)^3}{3!} + \frac{(i\theta)^4}{4!} + \frac{(i\theta)^5}{5!} + \cdots$$

$$= 1 + i\theta - \frac{\theta^2}{2!} - i\frac{\theta^3}{3!} + \frac{\theta^4}{4!} + i\frac{\theta^5}{5!} - \cdots$$

$$= \left[1 - \frac{\theta^2}{2!} + \frac{\theta^4}{4!} - \frac{\theta^6}{6!} + \cdots\right] + i \cdot \left[\theta - \frac{\theta^3}{3!} + \frac{\theta^5}{5!} - \cdots\right]$$

$$= \cos(\theta) + i \cdot \sin(\theta).$$

Euler's formula. The remarkable relationship

$$e^{i\theta} = \cos(\theta) + i \cdot \sin(\theta) \tag{4.4}$$

between an imaginary power of e and the sine and cosine functions is known as *Euler's formula* after its discoverer, Leonhard Euler (1707–1783).

Some examples of Euler's formula that are of special interest are

$$e^{i\pi} = \cos(\pi) + i\sin(\pi) = -1 + i(0) = -1 \,,$$
$$e^{i\pi/2} = \cos(\pi/2) + i\sin(\pi/2) = 0 + i(1) = i \,, \text{ and}$$
$$e^{2\pi i} = \cos(2\pi) + i\sin(2\pi) = 1 \,.$$

In general, for any real number θ, $\Re(e^{i\theta}) = \cos(\theta)$ and $\Im(e^{i\theta}) = \sin(\theta)$. Hence,

$$\left| e^{i\theta} \right| = \sqrt{\cos^2(\theta) + \sin^2(\theta)} = 1$$

regardless of the value of θ.

Geometrically, for real numbers r and θ, we get

$$re^{i\theta} = r(\cos(\theta) + i\sin(\theta)) = r\cos(\theta) + ir\sin(\theta)$$

so that the complex number $re^{i\theta}$ corresponds to the point in the xy-plane with Cartesian coordinates $(r\cos(\theta), r\sin(\theta))$. This same point has *polar coordinates* r and θ. For this reason, the form $re^{i\theta}$ is called the *polar form* of the complex number $r(\cos(\theta) + i\sin(\theta))$.

Observe that $\left| re^{i\theta} \right| = |r|$. So, $|r|$ is the modulus of $re^{i\theta}$. The number θ, viewed as an angle now, is called the *argument* of the complex number $re^{i\theta}$.

A simple computation shows that $(re^{i\theta}) \cdot (Re^{i\phi}) = r \cdot R \cdot e^{i(\theta + \phi)}$. Thus, when we multiply two complex numbers, expressed here in their polar forms, the modulus of the product is equal to the product of the individual moduli and the argument of the product is the *sum* of the individual arguments.

DeMoivre's law. When the equation $(e^{i\theta})^n = e^{in\theta}$ is translated into standard complex number form, we get

$$[\cos(\theta) + i\sin(\theta)]^n = \cos(n\theta) + i\sin(n\theta) \,. \tag{4.5}$$

This is called *DeMoivre's law*.

It is just a short step now to define the exponential function for every complex number. Namely, for any complex number $z = a + bi$,

$$e^z = e^{a+bi} = e^a \cdot e^{bi} = e^a \cdot (\cos(b) + i\sin(b)) \,. \tag{4.6}$$

The complex exponential function has many interesting and important properties, not least of which is that it is a conformal mapping. (See [18] and [46], for example.) For our purposes, the periodicity property of the exponential function is central.

4.3 Wave functions

Waves, periodicity, and frequency. For a fixed real number ω, the functions $t \mapsto \cos(\omega t)$ and $t \mapsto \sin(\omega t)$ have period $2\pi/\omega$ and frequency $\omega/(2\pi)$. If the value of ω is large, then these functions have high frequency and short wavelength; lower values of ω yield functions with longer waves and lower frequencies.

For a given real number ω, consider the function $E_\omega(t) = e^{i\omega t}$. Then

$$E_\omega(t + 2\pi/\omega) = e^{i\omega(t+2\pi/\omega)} = e^{i\omega t + 2\pi i} = e^{i\omega t} \cdot e^{2\pi i} = e^{i\omega t} = E_\omega(t),$$

where we have used the fact that $e^{2\pi i} = 1$. Thus, the function E_ω is *periodic* with period $2\pi/\omega$ and frequency $\omega/(2\pi)$.

Another point of view is to see that

$$E_\omega(t) = e^{i\omega t} = \cos(\omega t) + i\sin(\omega t)$$

which is a sum of two periodic functions each having period $2\pi/\omega$. So the sum also is periodic with that same period.

A signal, such as a radio, light, or sound wave, can, in principle, be decomposed into its components of specific frequencies. For example, we might try to decompose the sound wave from a musical instrument into the high notes, the mid-tones, bass, and so on. That is, a signal, viewed as a function propagated over time, might also be viewed as a composite of functions of the form $\cos(\omega t)$ and $\sin(\omega t)$, or, more compactly, $E_\omega(t) = e^{i\omega t}$, for various values of ω. The pertinent issue becomes how to determine which values of ω correspond to the different frequency components of a given signal $f(t)$, and, for each such ω, to find the amplitude of the associated component.

Fourier analysis. As a first step toward finding the different frequencies that make up a given signal, consider the "harmonic frequencies" $n/(2\pi)$ where n is an integer. The basic periodic functions having these frequencies are of the form $E_n(t) = e^{int}$. Two basic computations involving these functions are the following.

$$\text{For } m \neq n, \quad \int_0^{2\pi} e^{imt} \cdot e^{-int} \, dt = \int_0^{2\pi} e^{i(m-n)t} \, dt = \left. \frac{e^{i(m-n)t}}{i(m-n)} \right|_0^{2\pi} = 0,$$

since $e^{i(m-n)2\pi} = e^0 = 1$.

$$\text{For } m = n, \int_0^{2\pi} e^{int} \cdot e^{-int} \, dt = \int_0^{2\pi} e^0 \, dt = 2\pi \,.$$

These computations mean that, if a signal has the form

$$f(t) = \sum_{n \in \Lambda} c_n e^{int}$$

for integers n in some set Λ, then the amplitudes $\{c_n\}$ are given by

$$c_n = \frac{1}{2\pi} \int_0^{2\pi} f(t) \cdot e^{-int} \, dt \text{ for each } n \in \Lambda \,.$$

Applying this analysis to an arbitrary function f that is periodic on the interval $0 \le t \le 2\pi$, we *define* the n th Fourier coefficient of f by

$$\hat{f}(n) = \frac{1}{2\pi} \int_0^{2\pi} f(t) \cdot e^{-int} \, dt \,. \tag{4.7}$$

We have in mind that f somehow can be represented, at least on the interval $0 \le t \le 2\pi$, by the sum $\sum \hat{f}(n) e^{int}$. Determining precisely when such a representation is valid (and even what is meant by "representation" or "valid") is part of the subject of Fourier series, initiated in 1811 by Jean-Baptiste Joseph Fourier (1768–1830).

In our analysis of X-ray attenuation-coefficient functions, we will use a different tool, also pioneered by Fourier, called the *Fourier transform*. The Fourier transform is analogous to the Fourier series but it allows for all possible frequencies and does not assume that the signal is periodic.

4.4 Exercises

1. (a) Let z and w be complex numbers. Show that $\overline{(z + w)} = \overline{z} + \overline{w}$ and that $\overline{z \cdot w} = \overline{z} \cdot \overline{w}$.
   (b) Show that $\overline{re^{i\theta}} = re^{-i\theta}$.
   (c) Use (4.3) to express $\dfrac{1}{3 + 4i}$ in the form $a + bi$.

2. Evaluate the integral $\displaystyle\int_0^{2\pi} e^{i\theta} \, d\theta$.

3. (a) Show that $\displaystyle\int_0^{\infty} e^{-\lambda x} \cdot e^{-i\omega x} \, dx = \frac{\lambda - i\omega}{\lambda^2 + \omega^2}$, where λ and ω are real numbers with $\lambda > 0$.
   (b) Use part (a) to show that $\displaystyle\int_{-\infty}^{\infty} e^{-\lambda |x|} \cdot e^{-i\omega x} \, dx = \frac{2\lambda}{\lambda^2 + \omega^2}$.

4. (a) Use Euler's formula to show that

$$e^{-i\omega T} - e^{i\omega T} = -2i\sin(\omega T)$$

for all real numbers ω and T.

(b) Now show that $\displaystyle\int_{-T}^{T} e^{-i\omega x}\, dx = 2\,\frac{\sin(\omega T)}{\omega}$ for $\omega \neq 0$.

(c) Plot the graph of $S(\omega) = 2\,\dfrac{\sin(\omega T)}{\omega}$, as a function of the real variable ω, for $T = 1$, for $T = 0.5$, and for $T = 0.2$. (Note that setting $S(0) = 2T$ yields a continuous function on the real line.)

5. Use a change of variables to show that

$$\int_{-\infty}^{\infty} f(x - \alpha)\, e^{-i\omega x}\, dx = e^{-i\omega\alpha} \int_{-\infty}^{\infty} f(x)\, e^{-i\omega x}\, dx$$

for all real numbers ω and α.

6. (a) Show that the functions $F_1(t) = e^{(\alpha+\omega i)t}$ and $F_2(t) = e^{(\alpha-\omega i)t}$, where α and ω are real constants, satisfy the (second-order linear) differential equation

$$y'' - 2\alpha y' + (\alpha^2 + \omega^2)y = 0.$$

(b) Using Euler's formula, conclude that the functions $y_1 = e^{\alpha t}\cos(\omega t)$ and $y_2 = e^{\alpha t}\sin(\omega t)$ also satisfy the same differential equation. (In case $\alpha < 0$, these are examples of decaying wave functions.)

5

The Fourier Transform

5.1 Definition and examples

For a given function f such that $\int_{-\infty}^{\infty} |f(x)| \, dx < \infty$, the *Fourier transform* of f is defined, for each real number ω, by

$$\mathcal{F}f(\omega) := \int_{-\infty}^{\infty} f(x) \, e^{-i\omega x} \, dx. \tag{5.1}$$

The idea behind this definition is that, for each value of ω, the value of $\mathcal{F}f(\omega)$ captures the component of f that has the frequency $\omega/(2\pi)$ (and period $2\pi/\omega$).

Example 5.1. The Fourier transform of a Gaussian. Let $f(x) = e^{-Ax^2}$, for some positive constant $A > 0$. Then we have

$$\mathcal{F}f(\omega) = \sqrt{\frac{\pi}{A}} \, e^{-\frac{\omega^2}{4A}}. \tag{5.2}$$

To prove this, we first need the following fact.

Lemma 5.2. *For $A \neq 0$, we have $\int_{-\infty}^{\infty} e^{-Ax^2} \, dx = \sqrt{\frac{\pi}{A}}$.*

© Springer International Publishing Switzerland 2015
T.G. Feeman, *The Mathematics of Medical Imaging*, Springer Undergraduate
Texts in Mathematics and Technology, DOI 10.1007/978-3-319-22665-1_5

Proof. Squaring the integral, we get

$$\left(\int_{-\infty}^{\infty} e^{-Ax^2}\, dx\right)^2 = \left(\int_{-\infty}^{\infty} e^{-Ax^2}\, dx\right)\left(\int_{-\infty}^{\infty} e^{-Ax^2}\, dx\right)$$

$$= \left(\int_{-\infty}^{\infty} e^{-Ax^2}\, dx\right)\left(\int_{-\infty}^{\infty} e^{-Ay^2}\, dy\right)$$

$$= \int_{-\infty}^{\infty}\int_{-\infty}^{\infty} e^{-A(x^2+y^2)}\, dx\, dy$$

$$(\text{polar coordinates}) = \int_{\theta=0}^{2\pi}\int_{r=0}^{\infty} e^{-Ar^2}\, r\, dr\, d\theta$$

$$= \int_{\theta=0}^{2\pi}\left(\lim_{b\to\infty}\frac{1-e^{-Ab^2}}{2A}\right) d\theta$$

$$= \int_{\theta=0}^{2\pi}\frac{1}{2A}\, d\theta$$

$$= \frac{\pi}{A}\, .$$

Taking square roots proves the lemma.   □

Now to compute the Fourier transform for this example. For each ω,

$$\mathcal{F}f(\omega) = \int_{-\infty}^{\infty} e^{-Ax^2}\, e^{-i\omega x}\, dx$$

$$= \int_{-\infty}^{\infty} e^{-A(x^2+i\omega x/A)}\, dx$$

$$(\text{complete the square}) = \int_{-\infty}^{\infty} e^{-A(x^2+i\omega x/A+(i\omega/2A)^2)}\, e^{A(i\omega/2A)^2}\, dx$$

$$= e^{-\omega^2/4A}\int_{-\infty}^{\infty} e^{-A(x+i\omega/2A)^2}\, dx$$

$$= e^{-\omega^2/4A}\int_{-\infty}^{\infty} e^{-Au^2}\, du \ \text{ with } u = x + i\omega/2A$$

$$= \sqrt{\frac{\pi}{A}}\, e^{-\omega^2/4A} \ \text{ by the lemma.}$$

This establishes the result we were after.   □

Observe that if we take $A = 1/2$, then $f(x) = e^{-x^2/2}$ and $\mathcal{F}f(\omega) = \sqrt{2\pi}\, e^{-\omega^2/2}$, a constant multiple of f itself. In the language of linear algebra, this function f is an *eigenvector*, or *eigenfunction*, of the Fourier transform.

Additional examples are considered in the exercises. Let us look at some basic properties of the Fourier transform.

5.2 Properties and applications

Additivity. Because the integral of a sum of functions is equal to the sum of the integrals of the functions separately, it follows that

$$\mathcal{F}(f + g)(\omega) = \mathcal{F}f(\omega) + \mathcal{F}g(\omega) , \tag{5.3}$$

for all integrable functions f and g and every real number ω.

Constant multiples. Because the integral of $c \cdot f$ is equal to c times the integral of f, we see that

$$\mathcal{F}(cf)(\omega) = c \cdot \mathcal{F}f(\omega) , \tag{5.4}$$

for all integrable functions f, all (complex) numbers c, and every real number ω.

The two properties (5.3) and (5.4) taken together prove the following.

Proposition 5.3. *The Fourier transform acts as a linear transformation on the space of all absolutely integrable functions. That is, for two such functions f and g and any constants α and β, we get that*

$$\mathcal{F}(\alpha f + \beta g) = \alpha \mathcal{F}(f) + \beta \mathcal{F}(g). \tag{5.5}$$

Shifting/translation. For an integrable function f and fixed real number α, let $g(x) = f(x - \alpha)$. (So the graph of g is the graph of f shifted or translated to the right by α units.) Then

$$\mathcal{F}g(\omega) = e^{-i\omega\alpha} \mathcal{F}f(\omega). \tag{5.6}$$

Proof. For each ω, we get

$$\mathcal{F}g(\omega) = \int_{-\infty}^{\infty} f(x - \alpha) \, e^{-i\omega x} \, dx$$

$$(\text{let } u = x - \alpha) = \int_{-\infty}^{\infty} f(u) \, e^{-i\omega(u+\alpha)} \, du$$

$$= e^{-i\omega\alpha} \int_{-\infty}^{\infty} f(u) e^{-i\omega u} \, du$$

$$= e^{-i\omega\alpha} \, \mathcal{F}f(\omega) \quad \text{as claimed.}$$

$\square$

Since the graph of g is a simple translation of the graph of f, the magnitude of the component of g at any given frequency is the same as that of f. However, the components occur at different places in the two signals, so there is a phase shift or delay in the Fourier transform. Also, the fixed translation α encompasses more cycles of a wave at a higher frequency than at a lower one. (For instance, an interval of width $\alpha = 2\pi$ contains two cycles of the wave $y = \sin(2x)$, but only one cycle of the wave $y = \sin(x)$.) Therefore, the larger the value of α is relative to the wavelength $2\pi/\omega$ the larger will be the phase delay in the transform. That is, the phase delay in the transform is proportional to ω, which explains the factor of $e^{-i\omega\alpha}$ in the transform of the shifted function g.

Shifting/modulation. For a given function f and a fixed real number ω_0, let $h(x) = e^{i\omega_0 x} f(x)$. (So h "modulates" f by multiplying f by a periodic function of a fixed frequency $\omega_0/2\pi$.) Then

$$\mathcal{F}h(\omega) = \mathcal{F}f(\omega - \omega_0). \tag{5.7}$$

Proof. For each ω, we get

$$\mathcal{F}h(\omega) = \int_{-\infty}^{\infty} e^{i\omega_0 x} f(x) e^{-i\omega x} \, dx$$

$$= \int_{-\infty}^{\infty} f(x) e^{-i(\omega - \omega_0)x} \, dx$$

$$= \mathcal{F}f(\omega - \omega_0) \quad \text{(by definition!).}$$

$\square$

These two shifting properties show that a translation of f results in a modulation of $\mathcal{F}f$ while a modulation of f produces a translation of $\mathcal{F}f$.

Scaling. For a given function f and a fixed real number $a \neq 0$, let $\phi(x) = f(ax)$. Then

$$\mathcal{F}\phi(\omega) = \frac{1}{|a|} \mathcal{F}f(\omega/a). \tag{5.8}$$

Proof. Assume that $a > 0$ for now. For each ω, we get

$$\mathcal{F}\phi(\omega) = \int_{-\infty}^{\infty} f(ax)\, e^{-i\omega x}\, dx$$

$$(\text{let } u = ax) \;=\; \frac{1}{a} \int_{-\infty}^{\infty} f(u)\, e^{-i\omega u/a}\, du$$

$$= \frac{1}{a} \int_{-\infty}^{\infty} f(u)\, e^{-i(\omega/a)u}\, du$$

$$= \frac{1}{a}\mathcal{F}f(\omega/a) \quad \text{(by definition!)}.$$

A similar argument applies when $a < 0$. (Why do we get a factor of $1/|a|$ in this case?)

$\square$

Even and odd functions. A function f, defined on the real line, is *even* if $f(-x) = f(x)$ for every x. Similarly, a function g is *odd* if $g(-x) = -g(x)$ for every x. For example, the *cosine* function is even while the *sine* function is odd.

Using Euler's formula (4.4), $e^{i\theta} = \cos(\theta) + i\sin(\theta)$, we may write the Fourier transform of a suitable real-valued function f as

$$\mathcal{F}f(\omega) = \int_{-\infty}^{\infty} f(x)\cos(\omega x)\, dx - i \cdot \int_{-\infty}^{\infty} f(x)\sin(\omega x)\, dx.$$

Now, if f is even, then, for fixed ω, the function $x \mapsto f(x)\sin(\omega x)$ is odd, whence $\int_{-\infty}^{\infty} f(x)\sin(\omega x)\, dx = 0$. Thus, *an even function has a real-valued Fourier transform.*

Similarly, if f is odd, then $x \mapsto f(x)\cos(\omega x)$ is also odd for each fixed ω. Thus, $\int_{-\infty}^{\infty} f(x)\cos(\omega x)\, dx = 0$. It follows that *an odd function has a purely imaginary Fourier transform.*

Transform of the complex conjugate. For a complex-number-valued function f defined on the real line $\mathbb{R}$, the complex conjugate of f is the function $\bar{f}$ defined by

$$\bar{f}(x) = \overline{f(x)} \quad \text{for every real number } x. \tag{5.9}$$

To uncover the relationship between the Fourier transform of $\bar{f}$ and that of f, let ω be an arbitrary real number. Then we have

$$\mathcal{F}\bar{f}(\omega) = \int_{-\infty}^{\infty} \overline{f(x)}\, e^{-i\omega x}\, dx$$

$$= \int_{-\infty}^{\infty} \overline{f(x)}\, e^{i(-\omega)x}\, dx$$

$$= \int_{-\infty}^{\infty} \overline{f(x)\, e^{-i(-\omega)x}}\, dx$$

$$= \overline{\int_{-\infty}^{\infty} f(x)\, e^{-i(-\omega)x}\, dx}$$

$$= \overline{\mathcal{F}f(-\omega)}$$

$$= \overline{\mathcal{F}f(-\omega)}.$$

This proves the following proposition.

Proposition 5.4. *For an integrable function f defined on the real line, and for every real number ω,*

$$\mathcal{F}\bar{f}(\omega) = \overline{\mathcal{F}f(-\omega)}. \tag{5.10}$$

Example 5.5. Let $f(x) = \begin{cases} 1 & \text{if } -1 \le x \le 1, \\ 0 & \text{if } |x| > 1. \end{cases}$ Then the Fourier transform of f is $\mathcal{F}f(\omega) =$

$2\sin(\omega)/\omega$. Now let $\phi(x) = f(ax)$, where $a > 0$. That is, $\phi(x) = \begin{cases} 1 & \text{if } -1/a \le x \le 1/a, \\ 0 & \text{if } |x| > 1/a. \end{cases}$

So we already know from earlier work that $\mathcal{F}\phi(\omega) = 2\sin(\omega/a)/\omega$, which is the same as $(1/a)\mathcal{F}f(\omega/a)$. This agrees with the scaling result (5.8).

Example 5.6. Let $f(x) = \begin{cases} 1 & \text{if } -1 \le x \le 1, \\ 0 & \text{if } |x| > 1 \end{cases}$ as in the previous example. So, again, the Fourier transform of f is $\mathcal{F}f(\omega) = 2\sin(\omega)/\omega$. Now let

$$g(x) = f(x-2) = \begin{cases} 1 & \text{if } 1 \le x \le 3, \\ 0 & \text{if } x < 1 \text{ or } x > 3. \end{cases}$$

By the shifting/translation result (5.6), we get

$$\mathcal{F}g(\omega) = e^{-2i\omega}\mathcal{F}f(\omega) = 2e^{-2i\omega}\frac{\sin(\omega)}{\omega}.$$

Example 5.7. As an application of the shifting/modulation property (5.7), observe that

$$\cos(\omega_0 x) = (1/2)(e^{i\omega_0 x} + e^{-i\omega_0 x}).$$

Thus, for any suitable f, take $h(x) = f(x)\cos(\omega_0 x)$. That is,

$$h(x) = (1/2)e^{i\omega_0 x}f(x) + (1/2)e^{i(-\omega_0)x}f(x).$$

It follows that

$$\mathcal{F}h(\omega) = (1/2)\mathcal{F}f(\omega - \omega_0) + (1/2)\mathcal{F}f(\omega + \omega_0).$$

For a specific example, let $f(x) = \begin{cases} 1 \text{ if } -1 \le x \le 1, \\ 0 \quad \text{if } |x| > 1 \end{cases}$ as in the previous examples. So, again, the Fourier transform of f is $\mathcal{F}f(\omega) = 2\sin(\omega)/\omega$. With $h(x) = f(x)\cos(\omega_0 x)$, we get

$$\mathcal{F}h(\omega) = (1/2)\mathcal{F}f(\omega - \omega_0) + (1/2)\mathcal{F}f(\omega + \omega_0)$$
$$= (1/2)\left\{ 2\frac{\sin(\omega - \omega_0)}{(\omega - \omega_0)} + 2\frac{\sin(\omega + \omega_0)}{(\omega + \omega_0)} \right\}$$
$$= \frac{\sin(\omega - \omega_0)}{(\omega - \omega_0)} + \frac{\sin(\omega + \omega_0)}{(\omega + \omega_0)}$$

The graph of $\mathcal{F}f$ in this example has a main peak of height 2 centered at $\omega = 0$ with smaller ripples at the edges. The graph of $\mathcal{F}h$ has two main peaks, centered at $\omega = \pm\omega_0$, with a valley in between and smaller ripples at the edges.

5.3 Heaviside and Dirac δ

Definition 5.8. The *Heaviside function* H is defined by

$$H(x) = \begin{cases} 0 \text{ if } x < 0, \\ 1 \text{ if } x > 0. \end{cases} \tag{5.11}$$

Technically, $H(0)$ is not defined, which, nonetheless, does not stop us from writing formulas like

$$H(x - a) - H(x - b) = \begin{cases} 1 \text{ if } a < x < b, \\ 0 \quad \text{otherwise.} \end{cases}$$

Definition 5.9. The *Dirac δ function*, denoted simply by δ, is defined to be the formal derivative $\delta = dH/dx$ of the Heaviside function with respect to x.

Of course, since H is constant except at 0, we get that $\delta(x) = 0$ except at $x = 0$ where H does not have a derivative (or the derivative is essentially ∞). So apparently $\delta(0)$ does not make sense. Alternatively, we can think of $\delta(0)$ as being equal to ∞. So the "graph" of δ basically consists of an infinitely tall spike at 0. (*Warning:* We should not expect a computer to plot this graph for us!) The Dirac δ function is also known as the *impulse function*, perhaps because its graph (!) evokes the image of a sudden massive impulse of energy that immediately dies out again.

Neither H nor δ can exist in reality as a physical signal. The Heaviside signal would have to appear out of nowhere (like a Big Bang?) and then propagate without loss of energy for eternity. The δ impulse also would have to appear out of nowhere, but then die instantly. Moreover, neither of these functions is even properly defined as a *function*. Instead, they fall into a class known as *generalized functions* or *distributions*. Nonetheless, they are useful idealized mathematical and physical constructs and we shall use them without further troubling ourselves over their precise natures.

Integrals involving H and δ. In the context of integration, the Heaviside function has a property of central importance. Formally, the value of H jumps by 1 at 0; so we can think of the differential dH as having the value 1 at 0 and the value 0 everywhere else. This point of view suggests that

$$\int_{-\infty}^{\infty} f(x)\, dH = f(0) \tag{5.12}$$

for any function f. The intuitive idea here is that dH is 0 except at 0 where $dH = 1$, so the value of the integral is just $f(0) \cdot 1 = f(0)$. In fact, this is an example of a theory of integrals known as *Riemann–Stieltjes integration* that generalizes the sort of integration we typically learn in a first course in calculus. For our purposes here, we will simply accept this integral as a defining feature of the Heaviside function.

Next, since $\delta = dH/dx$, it follows that $dH = \delta(x)\, dx$. Hence, for any f, it follows from (5.12) that

$$\int_{-\infty}^{\infty} f(x)\delta(x)\, dx = \int_{-\infty}^{\infty} f(x)\, dH = f(0). \tag{5.13}$$

This integral formula will feature prominently in what lies ahead for us.

For a first example, substitute the constant function $f(x) = 1$ into (5.13). This yields the formula

$$\int_{-\infty}^{\infty} \delta(x)\, dx = 1. \tag{5.14}$$

Thus, the graph of δ is an infinitely tall spike with no width but which has "underneath it" an area of 1! This truly is a strange function.

As a generalization of formula (5.13), we have the following result, whose proof is left as an exercise.

$$\text{For } a \in \mathbb{R}, \ \int_{-\infty}^{\infty} f(x)\delta(x - a)\, dx = f(a). \tag{5.15}$$

Remark 5.10. There are other ways of thinking about δ. For instance, the equation (5.21) below can be taken as a definition, with Lemma 5.13 providing the justification. Alternatively, we can define the δ function as a limit by setting

$$\delta(x) = \lim_{a \to 0^+} \left(\frac{1}{2a}\right) \sqcap_a (x), \tag{5.16}$$

where $\Pi_a(x) = \begin{cases} 1 & \text{if } -a \leq x \leq a, \\ 0 & \text{if } |x| > a. \end{cases}$ We will take advantage of this approach in Chapter 7.

(The function Π_a is also called the *characteristic function* of the interval $[-a, a]$ and is often denoted by $\chi_{[-a, a]}$. We will use the symbol Π to remind us of the shape of its graph.)

$\mathcal{F}$ **and δ.** We use (5.13) to compute the Fourier transform of the δ function. Namely,

$$\mathcal{F}\delta(\omega) = \int_{-\infty}^{\infty} \delta(x)\, e^{-i\omega x}\, dx = e^{-i\omega \cdot 0} = e^0 = 1. \tag{5.17}$$

So the Fourier transform of δ is the constant function equal to 1.

5.4 Inversion of the Fourier transform

In the definition of the Fourier transform (5.1), there may seem to be no reason *a priori* to have used the exponent $-i\omega x$ rather than its opposite $+i\omega x$. This prompts the following definition.

Definition 5.11. For a function g for which $\int_{-\infty}^{\infty} |g(\omega)|\, d\omega < \infty$, the *inverse Fourier transform* of g is defined, for each real number x, by

$$\mathcal{F}^{-1} g(x) := \frac{1}{2\pi} \int_{\omega=-\infty}^{\infty} g(\omega)\, e^{i\omega x}\, d\omega. \tag{5.18}$$

The reasons for the factor $1/2\pi$ as well as for the name of this transform are made clear by the following essential theorem.

Theorem 5.12. Fourier inversion theorem. *If f is continuous on the real line and $\int_{-\infty}^{\infty} |f(x)|\, dx < \infty$, then*

$$\mathcal{F}^{-1}(\mathcal{F}f)(x) = f(x) \quad \text{for all } x. \tag{5.19}$$

To prove this, we first need a lemma.

Lemma 5.13. *For real numbers t and x,*

$$\int_{\omega=-\infty}^{\infty} e^{i\omega(t-x)}\, d\omega = \lim_{\varepsilon \to 0} \sqrt{\frac{\pi}{\varepsilon}} \cdot e^{-(x-t)^2/(4\varepsilon)}. \tag{5.20}$$

Proof of Lemma 5.13. For each real number ω we have $\lim_{\varepsilon \to 0} e^{-\varepsilon \omega^2} = 1$. Thus, for any real numbers t and x,

$$\int_{\omega=-\infty}^{\infty} e^{i\omega(t-x)}\, d\omega = \lim_{\varepsilon \to 0} \int_{\omega=-\infty}^{\infty} e^{-\varepsilon \omega^2} \cdot e^{i\omega(t-x)}\, d\omega$$

$$= \lim_{\varepsilon \to 0} \int_{\omega=-\infty}^{\infty} e^{-\varepsilon \omega^2} \cdot e^{-i\omega(x-t)}\, d\omega.$$

Previously, we computed the Fourier transform of a Gaussian function e^{-Ax^2} to be $\sqrt{\pi/A}\,e^{-t^2/(4A)}$. Applying this formula to the Gaussian function $e^{-\varepsilon\omega^2}$ (so $A = \varepsilon$ and ω is in place of x) and evaluating the resulting Fourier transform at $(x - t)$ yields

$$\int_{\omega=-\infty}^{\infty} e^{-\varepsilon\omega^2} \cdot e^{-i\omega(x-t)}\, d\omega = \sqrt{\frac{\pi}{\varepsilon}}\, e^{-(x-t)^2/(4\varepsilon)}.$$

Substituting this into the previous calculation, we get

$$\int_{\omega=-\infty}^{\infty} e^{i\omega(t-x)}\, d\omega = \lim_{\varepsilon\to 0} \int_{\omega=-\infty}^{\infty} e^{-\varepsilon\omega^2} \cdot e^{-i\omega(x-t)}\, d\omega$$

$$= \lim_{\varepsilon\to 0} \sqrt{\frac{\pi}{\varepsilon}}\, e^{-(x-t)^2/(4\varepsilon)},$$

which establishes the lemma.   □

Proof of Theorem 5.12. For a continuous function f that is absolutely integrable on the real line, let F denote the Fourier transform $\mathcal{F}f$. For any real number t, we get

$$\mathcal{F}^{-1}F(t) = \frac{1}{2\pi} \int_{\omega=-\infty}^{\infty} F(\omega)\, e^{i\omega t}\, d\omega$$

$$= \frac{1}{2\pi} \int_{\omega=-\infty}^{\infty} \int_{x=-\infty}^{\infty} f(x)\, e^{-i\omega x}\, e^{i\omega t}\, dx\, d\omega \text{ (by definition of } F)$$

$$= \frac{1}{2\pi} \int_{x=-\infty}^{\infty} \int_{\omega=-\infty}^{\infty} f(x)\, e^{i\omega(t-x)}\, d\omega\, dx$$

$$= \frac{1}{2\pi} \int_{x=-\infty}^{\infty} f(x) \left(\int_{\omega=-\infty}^{\infty} e^{i\omega(t-x)}\, d\omega \right) dx$$

$$= \frac{1}{2\pi} \cdot \lim_{\varepsilon\to 0} \int_{x=-\infty}^{\infty} f(x) \sqrt{\frac{\pi}{\varepsilon}}\, e^{-(x-t)^2/(4\varepsilon)}\, dx \text{ (by the lemma).}$$

Set $y = (x - t)/(2\sqrt{\varepsilon})$, so $x = t + 2\sqrt{\varepsilon}y$ and $dx = 2\sqrt{\varepsilon}\, dy$:

$$\mathcal{F}^{-1}F(t) = \frac{1}{2\pi} \cdot \lim_{\varepsilon\to 0} \left(\sqrt{\frac{\pi}{\varepsilon}} \cdot 2\sqrt{\varepsilon} \right) \int_{y=-\infty}^{\infty} f(t + 2\sqrt{\varepsilon}y)\, e^{-y^2}\, dy$$

$$= \frac{1}{\sqrt{\pi}} \cdot f(t) \cdot \int_{y=-\infty}^{\infty} e^{-y^2}\, dy \text{ (since } \lim_{\varepsilon\to 0} f(t + 2\sqrt{\varepsilon}y) = f(t)\forall y)$$

$$= \frac{1}{\sqrt{\pi}} \cdot f(t) \cdot \sqrt{\pi}$$

$$= f(t).$$

This is the desired result.   □

A bit more generally, if f has a point of discontinuity at α and if the one-sided limits $\lim_{x \to \alpha-} f(x)$ and $\lim_{x \to \alpha+} f(x)$ both exist, then

$$\mathcal{F}^{-1}(\mathcal{F}f)(\alpha) = (1/2) \left(\lim_{x \to \alpha-} f(x) + \lim_{x \to \alpha+} f(x) \right).$$

The proof of this claim is left as an exercise.

Example 5.14. Right away let's apply the inverse Fourier transform to a function that is not even a function! We saw before that the Fourier transform of the δ function is the constant function to 1. That means that the δ function is the inverse Fourier transform of the constant function 1. That is,

$$\delta(x) = \mathcal{F}^{-1}1(x) = \frac{1}{2\pi} \int_{-\infty}^{\infty} e^{i\omega x} \, d\omega \tag{5.21}$$

for all x. Interestingly, had we elected to *define* the δ function by this integral, then we could have used that to provide a simpler proof of the Fourier inversion theorem, Theorem 5.12. (See (2.12) in [9].)

Example 5.15. Inverse Fourier transform of a Gaussian. We have already seen that the Fourier transform of a Gaussian is another Gaussian. Thus, the same will be true for the inverse Fourier transform of a Gaussian. Specifically,

$$\mathcal{F}^{-1}(e^{-B\omega^2})(x) = \frac{1}{2\pi} \int_{-\infty}^{\infty} e^{-B\omega^2} e^{i\omega x} \, d\omega$$

$$= \sqrt{\frac{1}{4\pi B}} e^{-x^2/(4B)} . \tag{5.22}$$

In particular, if we take $B = 1/(4A)$ and multiply both sides by $\sqrt{\pi/A}$ we see that we get e^{-Ax^2}, illustrating again the inverse relationship between the transforms (5.1) and (5.18).

Example 5.16. Inverse Fourier transform of a square wave. As in (5.16), let

$$\Pi_a(x) = \begin{cases} 1 & \text{if } -a \le x \le a, \\ 0 & \text{if } |x| > a. \end{cases} \tag{5.23}$$

Then the inverse Fourier transform of Π_a is given by

$$\mathcal{F}^{-1} \Pi_a(x) = \frac{1}{2\pi} \int_{\omega=-\infty}^{\infty} \Pi_a(\omega) e^{i\omega x} \, d\omega$$

$$= \frac{1}{2\pi} \int_{\omega=-a}^{a} e^{i\omega x} \, d\omega$$

$$= \frac{1}{2\pi} \frac{e^{iax} - e^{-iax}}{ix}$$

$$= \frac{1}{\pi} \frac{\sin(ax)}{x} , \qquad (5.24)$$

where Euler's formula (4.4) was used in the final step.

5.5 Multivariable forms

We will need two generalizations of the Fourier transform in order to apply it within the context of medical imaging, where the functions involved are defined in the plane using either Cartesian or polar coordinates.

First, for a function $h(r, \theta)$ defined using polar coordinates in the plane, we simply apply the one-variable Fourier transform in the radial variable (r) only. This gives the following definitions.

Definition 5.17. For $h(r, \theta)$, we define the Fourier transform of h at a point (t, θ) (also in polar coordinates and with the same angle θ) by

$$\mathcal{F}h(t, \theta) = \int_{r=-\infty}^{\infty} h(r, \theta) e^{-irt} dr . \qquad (5.25)$$

Definition 5.18. Similarly, the inverse Fourier transform of h is given by

$$\mathcal{F}^{-1}h(t, \theta) = \frac{1}{2\pi} \int_{r=-\infty}^{\infty} h(r, \theta) e^{irt} dr . \qquad (5.26)$$

The inverse relationship between these transforms is clear because the variable θ is treated as a constant in the computations. Significantly, this generalization of the Fourier transform and its inverse applies to the Radon transform of a function f since $\mathcal{R}f$ is defined at the points (t, θ) corresponding to the lines $\ell_{t, \theta}$.

The second generalization of the Fourier transform is applied to functions g defined using Cartesian coordinates in the plane. For instance, $g(x, y)$ might represent the X-ray attenuation coefficient of a tissue sample located at the point (x, y).

Definition 5.19. For such a function g, we define the Fourier transform of g evaluated at the point (X, Y) (also in Cartesian coordinates in the plane) by

$$\mathcal{F}g(X, Y) = \int_{-\infty}^{\infty} \int_{-\infty}^{\infty} g(x, y)) e^{-i(xX+yY)} dx \, dy. \qquad (5.27)$$

Definition 5.20. Similarly, the inverse Fourier transform of g at (x, y) is given by

$$\mathcal{F}^{-1}g(x, y) = \frac{1}{4\pi^2} \int_{-\infty}^{\infty} \int_{-\infty}^{\infty} g(X, Y) \, e^{i(xX+yY)} \, dX \, dY. \tag{5.28}$$

As in the one-variable setting, we have the inverse relationship

$$\mathcal{F}^{-1}(\mathcal{F}g)(x, y) = \mathcal{F}(\mathcal{F}^{-1}g)(x, y) = g(x, y).$$

Of course, some assumptions and restrictions on g are necessary for these integrals to make sense, but we will gloss over these concerns here. (See Appendix A for details.)

A geometric viewpoint. Consider a vector $\langle X, Y \rangle = \langle r\cos(\theta), r\sin(\theta) \rangle$ in $\mathbb{R}^2$. For arbitrary real numbers x and y, let

$$t = x\cos(\theta) + y\sin(\theta),$$
$$s = -x\sin(\theta) + y\cos(\theta), \text{ and}$$
$$\langle x_1, y_1 \rangle = \langle -s\sin(\theta), s\cos(\theta) \rangle.$$

Then

$$\langle x, y \rangle = \langle t\cos(\theta), t\sin(\theta) \rangle + \langle x_1, y_1 \rangle,$$

and, because $\langle x_1, y_1 \rangle \bullet \langle \cos(\theta), \sin(\theta) \rangle = 0$, it follows that

$$xX + yY = rt\cos^2(\theta) + rt\sin^2(\theta) + r(x_1\cos(\theta) + y_1\sin(\theta)) = rt.$$

Thus, the expression $e^{-i(xX+yY)}$ in the definition of the 2-dimensional Fourier transform is the same as the expression e^{-irt} that appears in the one-variable Fourier transform. This function is periodic with period $2\pi/r$ but, in this setting, adding a multiple of $2\pi/r$ to the value of t amounts to moving the point (x, y) by a distance of $2\pi/r$ in the direction of the vector $\langle \cos(\theta), \sin(\theta) \rangle$. In other words, the function $e^{-i(xX+yY)}$ oscillates with period $2\pi/\sqrt{X^2 + Y^2} \, (= 2\pi/r)$ in the direction of the vector $\langle X, Y \rangle$.

In higher dimensions, suppose the function g is defined in n-dimensional space and represent points in n-dimensional space as vectors, such as $\mathbf{u}$ or $\mathbf{v}$. The n-dimensional Fourier transform is defined by

$$\mathcal{F}g(\mathbf{u}) = \int_{\mathbb{R}^n} g(\mathbf{v}) \, e^{-i(\mathbf{u} \bullet \mathbf{v})} \, d\mathbf{v}. \tag{5.29}$$

We will not have occasion to use the generalized Fourier transform for $n > 2$.

The Dirac δ function can also be defined as a function in the plane. Using Cartesian coordinates, we set

$$\delta(x, y) = \delta(x) \cdot \delta(y).$$ (5.30)

Observe that

$$\int\int_{x,y=-\infty}^{\infty} \delta(x, y)\, dx\, dy = \left(\int_{x=-\infty}^{\infty} \delta(x)\, dx\right) \cdot \left(\int_{y=-\infty}^{\infty} \delta(y)\, dy\right) = 1 \cdot 1 = 1,$$

as required.

For polar coordinates, as with the Fourier transform, we interpret δ as depending only on the radial variable. Since we require the integral of δ over the plane to have the value 1, and the change of coordinates in the plane is $dx\, dy = r\, dr\, d\theta$, we now define

$$\delta(r, \theta) = \frac{1}{\pi r}\delta(r).$$ (5.31)

With this definition, when we integrate over the plane, we get

$$\int_{\theta=0}^{\pi}\int_{r=-\infty}^{\infty} \delta(r, \theta)\, r\, dr\, d\theta = \int_{r=-\infty}^{\infty} \delta(r)\, dr = 1,$$

as required.

For either choice of coordinates, the 2-D δ function may be viewed as a limit by setting

$$\delta(r) = \lim_{a\to 0+} \begin{cases} \frac{1}{2a} & \text{if } -a \le r \le a, \\ 0 & \text{if } |r| > a. \end{cases}$$ (5.32)

5.6 Exercises

1. Use the shifting rules, (5.6) and (5.7), to examine the following examples. (In each case, the Fourier transform of the given function has been computed previously.)

(a) Let $f(x) = e^{-|x|}$. Then the Fourier transform of f is

$$\mathcal{F}f(\omega) = \frac{2}{1 + \omega^2}.$$

(i)   Compute the Fourier transform of $g(x) = f(x - \alpha)$, where α is a constant;

(ii)   Compute the Fourier transform of $h(x) = e^{i\omega_0 x} f(x)$,
where ω_0 is a constant;

(iii)   Plot the Fourier transform of f, the Fourier transform of g with $\alpha = 1$, and the Fourier transform of h with $\omega_0 = \pi/2$.

(b)   For $\sqcap_{1/2}(x) = \begin{cases} 1 \text{ if } -\frac{1}{2} \le x \le \frac{1}{2}, \\ 0 \quad \text{if } |x| > \frac{1}{2}, \end{cases}$ the Fourier transform is

$$\mathcal{F}\sqcap_{1/2}(\omega) = \frac{\sin(\omega/2)}{(\omega/2)}.$$

(i)   Compute the Fourier transform of $g(x) = \sqcap_{1/2}(x - \alpha)$,
where α is a constant;

(ii)   Compute the Fourier transform of $h(x) = e^{i\omega_0 x} \sqcap_{1/2}(x)$,
where ω_0 is a constant;

(iii)   Plot the Fourier transform of $\sqcap_{1/2}$, the Fourier transform of g with $\alpha = 1$, and the Fourier transform of h with $\omega_0 = \pi/2$.

(c)   For $f(x) := e^{-x^2/2}$, the Fourier transform of f is

$$\mathcal{F}f(\omega) = \sqrt{2\pi}\, e^{-\omega^2/2}.$$

(i)   Compute the Fourier transform of $g(x) = f(x - \alpha)$,
where α is a constant;

(ii)   Compute the Fourier transform of $h(x) = e^{i\omega_0 x} f(x)$,
where ω_0 is a constant;

(iii)   Plot the Fourier transform of f, the Fourier transform of g with $\alpha = 1$, and the Fourier transform of h with $\omega_0 = \pi/2$.

2.   Recall Euler's Formula: $e^{it} = \cos(t) + i\sin(t)$ for every real number t.

(a)   Prove that $\cos(ax) = \left(e^{iax} + e^{-iax}\right)/2$ for all real numbers a and x.

(b)   Prove that the function $G(x) = e^{iax}$ has period $2\pi/a$.

(c)   Explain, based on parts (a) and (b), why the Fourier transform of $f(x) = \cos(ax)$ consists of two impulses, located at the values $\omega = \pm a$ corresponding to the frequencies $\pm\dfrac{a}{2\pi}$.

3.   With the assumption that $\lim_{x \to \pm\infty} f(x)\, e^{-i\omega x} = 0$ for all ω, show that

$$\mathcal{F}(f')(\omega) = i\omega\,\mathcal{F}f(\omega) \text{ for all } \omega.$$

4. Again using the fact that $F(\omega) = \dfrac{2}{1+\omega^2}$ is the Fourier transform of $f(x) = e^{-|x|}$, compute the inverse Fourier transform of

$$H(\omega) = \frac{1}{1 + B^2(\omega - \omega_0)^2},$$

where B and ω_0 are (real) constants. (Such a function H is called a *Lorentzian*.)

5. A common type of signal is a *decaying wave*. Compute the Fourier transforms of the following two decaying waves. (Assume that $\lambda > 0$ in both cases.)

   (a) (two-way decaying wave) $f(x) = e^{-\lambda|x|} \cos(\omega_0 x)$;

   (b) (one-way decaying wave) $g(x) = \begin{cases} e^{-\lambda x} \cos(\omega_0 x) & \text{if } x \geq 0, \\ 0 & \text{if } x < 0. \end{cases}$

6. Provide a proof of the integral formula (5.15): For $a \in \mathbb{R}$,

$$\int_{-\infty}^{\infty} f(x)\delta(x - a) \, dx = f(a). \tag{5.33}$$

7. Show that the inverse Fourier transform of an even function is a real-valued function while the inverse Fourier transform of an odd function is purely imaginary (has real part equal to 0).

8. Let f be absolutely integrable on the real line and piecewise continuous with a point of discontinuity at α. In particular, the one-sided limits $\lim_{x\to\alpha^-} f(x)$ and $\lim_{x\to\alpha^+} f(x)$ both exist. Prove that

$$\mathcal{F}^{-1}(\mathcal{F}f)(\alpha) = (1/2) \left(\lim_{x\to\alpha^-} f(x) + \lim_{x\to\alpha^+} f(x) \right).$$

6

Two Big Theorems

The ideas discussed in this chapter involve interactions between three transforms — the Radon transform, the Fourier transform, and the back-projection transform. Each of these transforms is defined in terms of improper integrals on infinite intervals. This raises the somewhat technical matter of determining which functions may appropriately be considered, an issue that is addressed in Appendix A. For the time being, we assume that any function being considered here meets the requirements. For those functions that arise in the practical world of medical imaging this is certainly the case.

6.1 The central slice theorem

The interaction between the Fourier transform and the Radon transform is expressed in an equation known as the *central slice theorem* (also called the *central projection theorem*).

In this presentation, the symbols $\mathcal{F}$ and $\mathcal{F}_2$ are used to denote the 1- and 2-dimensional Fourier transforms, respectively. The Radon transform is denoted by $\mathcal{R}$. The function f, representing, say, an X-ray attenuation coefficient, is a function of 2-dimensional Cartesian coordinates.

Theorem 6.1. Central slice theorem. *For any suitable function f defined in the plane and all real numbers S and θ,*

$$\mathcal{F}_2 f(S\cos(\theta), S\sin(\theta)) = \mathcal{F}(\mathcal{R}f)(S, \theta). \tag{6.1}$$

Proof. Given f defined in the plane and real numbers S and θ, the definition of the 2-dimensional Fourier transform gives

$$\mathcal{F}_2 f(S\cos(\theta), S\sin(\theta)) = \int_{-\infty}^{\infty} \int_{-\infty}^{\infty} f(x, y) \, e^{-iS(x\cos(\theta)+y\sin(\theta))} \, dx\, dy. \tag{6.2}$$

© Springer International Publishing Switzerland 2015
T.G. Feeman, *The Mathematics of Medical Imaging*, Springer Undergraduate
Texts in Mathematics and Technology, DOI 10.1007/978-3-319-22665-1_6

Now, instead of integrating separately over $-\infty < x < \infty$ and $-\infty < y < \infty$, we can reorganize the points in the xy-plane according to the value of $x\cos(\theta)+y\sin(\theta)$. Specifically, for each real number t, gather together all of the points (x, y) in the plane for which $x\cos(\theta)+y\sin(\theta) = t$. *This is exactly the line $\ell_{t,\theta}$!* From our earlier analysis, we know that, for each point (x, y) on $\ell_{t,\theta}$, the real number $s = -x\sin(\theta)+y\cos(\theta)$ satisfies $x = t\cos(\theta) - s\sin(\theta)$ and $y = t\sin(\theta) + s\cos(\theta)$. Moreover, the matrix $\begin{bmatrix} \partial x/\partial t & \partial x/\partial s \\ \partial y/\partial t & \partial y/\partial s \end{bmatrix}$ has determinant 1, so that $ds\,dt = dx\,dy$ when the change of variables is put in place. With these changes, the right-hand side of (6.2) becomes

$$\int_{-\infty}^{\infty} \int_{-\infty}^{\infty} f(t\cos(\theta) - s\sin(\theta),\, t\sin(\theta) + s\cos(\theta))\, e^{-iSt}\, ds\, dt. \tag{6.3}$$

The factor e^{-iSt} in the integrand of (6.3) does not depend on s, so it may be factored out of the inner integral. Thus, (6.3) becomes

$$\int_{-\infty}^{\infty} \left(\int_{-\infty}^{\infty} f(t\cos(\theta) - s\sin(\theta),\, t\sin(\theta) + s\cos(\theta))\, ds \right) e^{-iSt}\, dt. \tag{6.4}$$

The inner integral in (6.4) is exactly the definition of $\mathcal{R}f(t, \theta)$, the Radon transform of the function f evaluated at the point (t, θ). That is, (6.4) is the same as

$$\int_{-\infty}^{\infty} (\mathcal{R}f(t, \theta))\, e^{-iSt}\, dt. \tag{6.5}$$

Finally, the integral (6.5) is the definition of the Fourier transform of $\mathcal{R}f$ evaluated at (S, θ). That is, (6.5) is equal to

$$\mathcal{F}(\mathcal{R}f)(S, \theta). \tag{6.6}$$

We have established, as we set out to do, the equality

$$\mathcal{F}_2 f(S\cos(\theta), S\sin(\theta)) = \mathcal{F}(\mathcal{R}f)(S, \theta). \tag{6.7}$$

$\square$

6.2 Filtered back projection

The back projection served as a first attempt at inverting the Radon transform and recovering the X-ray attenuation-coefficient function. The result was not the original function but a smoothed-out version of it. The next theorem, called the *filtered back-projection formula*, shows how to correct for the smoothing effect and recover the original function.

Theorem 6.2. The filtered back-projection formula. *For a suitable function f defined in the plane and real numbers x and y,*

$$f(x, y) = \frac{1}{2} \mathcal{B} \left\{ \mathcal{F}^{-1} \left[|S| \, \mathcal{F} \left(\mathcal{R}f \right) (S, \, \theta) \right] \right\} (x, \, y). \tag{6.8}$$

Proof. The (2-dimensional) Fourier transform and its inverse transform are just that — inverses. Hence, for any suitable function f and any point (x, y) in the plane, we get

$$f(x, y) = \mathcal{F}_2^{-1} \mathcal{F}_2 f(x, y). \tag{6.9}$$

Applying the definition of the inverse 2-dimensional Fourier transform, the right-hand side of (6.9) becomes

$$\frac{1}{4\pi^2} \int_{-\infty}^{\infty} \int_{-\infty}^{\infty} \mathcal{F}_2 f(X, \, Y) \, e^{+i(xX + yY)} \, dX \, dY. \tag{6.10}$$

Now change variables from Cartesian coordinates $(X, \, Y)$ to polar coordinates $(S, \, \theta)$, where $X = S \cos(\theta)$ and $Y = S \sin(\theta)$. Rather than use the usual intervals $0 \leq S < \infty$ and $0 \leq \theta \leq 2\pi$, however, allow S to be any real number and restrict θ to $0 \leq \theta \leq \pi$. With this variation, we get $dX \, dY = |S| \, dS \, d\theta$ (rather than $S \, dS \, d\theta$). With these changes, (6.10) becomes

$$\frac{1}{4\pi^2} \int_0^{\pi} \int_{-\infty}^{\infty} \mathcal{F}_2 f(S \cos(\theta), \, S \sin(\theta)) \, e^{+iS(x \cos(\theta) + y \sin(\theta))} \, |S| \, dS \, d\theta. \tag{6.11}$$

The factor $\mathcal{F}_2 f(S \cos(\theta), \, S \sin(\theta))$ in the integrand of (6.11) is, according to the central slice theorem (Theorem 6.1), the same as $\mathcal{F} \left(\mathcal{R}f \right) (S, \, \theta)$. Thus, (6.11) is the same as

$$\frac{1}{4\pi^2} \int_0^{\pi} \int_{-\infty}^{\infty} \mathcal{F} \left(\mathcal{R}f \right) (S, \, \theta) \, e^{+iS(x \cos(\theta) + y \sin(\theta))} \, |S| \, dS \, d\theta. \tag{6.12}$$

The inner integral (with respect to S) in (6.12) is, by definition, 2π times the inverse Fourier transform of the function $|S| \, \mathcal{F} \left(\mathcal{R}f \right) (S, \, \theta)$ evaluated at the point $(x \cos(\theta) + y \sin(\theta), \, \theta)$. That is, (6.12) is the same as

$$\frac{1}{2\pi} \int_0^{\pi} \mathcal{F}^{-1} \left[|S| \, \mathcal{F} \left(\mathcal{R}f \right) (S, \, \theta) \right] (x \cos(\theta) + y \sin(\theta), \, \theta) \, d\theta. \tag{6.13}$$

Finally, the integral in (6.13) is the one used in the back projection of the (admittedly somewhat elaborate) function $\mathcal{F}^{-1} \left[|S| \, \mathcal{F} \left(\mathcal{R}f \right) (S, \, \theta) \right]$. Hence, (6.13) is equal to

$$\frac{1}{2} \mathcal{B} \left\{ \mathcal{F}^{-1} \left[|S| \, \mathcal{F} \left(\mathcal{R}f \right) (S, \, \theta) \right] \right\} (x, \, y). \tag{6.14}$$

We have successfully established the desired formula

$$f(x, y) = \frac{1}{2} \mathcal{B} \left\{ \mathcal{F}^{-1} \left[|S| \, \mathcal{F} \left(\mathcal{R}f \right) (S, \theta) \right] \right\} (x, y). \tag{6.15}$$

$\square$

Without the factor of $|S|$ in the formula, the Fourier transform and its inverse would cancel out and the result would be simply the back projection of the Radon transform of f, which we know does not lead to recovery of f. Thus, the essential element in the formula is to multiply the Fourier transform of $\mathcal{R}f(S, \theta)$ by the absolute-value function $|S|$ *before* the inverse Fourier transform is applied. In the language of signal processing, we say that the Fourier transform of $\mathcal{R}f$ is *filtered* by multiplication by $|S|$. That is why the formula is called the filtered back-projection formula. We will discuss filters in greater detail in the next chapter.

The filtered back-projection formula is the fundamental basis for image reconstruction. However, it assumes that the values of $\mathcal{R}f(S, \theta)$ are known for all possible lines $\ell_{S,\theta}$. In practice, of course, this is not the case. Only a finite number of X-ray samples are taken and we must approximate an image from the resulting data. Indeed, for any finite set of X-rays that make up a scan, there will be so-called *ghosts*: nonzero attenuation coefficient functions whose Radon transforms vanish on all lines in the scan. For instance, try to imagine a function that is nonzero only in the gaps between the lines in Figure 1.2! See [36] for more about ghosts.

Soon, we will turn our attention to the practical implementation of the filtered back-projection formula. But first, let us look at a different formula for recovering f that was presented by Radon in 1917 ([43]).

6.3 The Hilbert transform

A property of the Fourier transform that was addressed in Chapter 5, in Exercise 3, concerns the interaction of the Fourier transform with the derivative of a function. To wit,

$$\mathcal{F}\left(\frac{df}{dx}\right)(\omega) = i\omega \, \mathcal{F}(f)(\omega). \tag{6.16}$$

Applied to the Radon transform, (6.16) yields

$$\mathcal{F}\left(\frac{\partial (\mathcal{R}f)(t, \theta)}{\partial t}\right)(S, \theta) = iS \, \mathcal{F}(\mathcal{R}f)(S, \theta). \tag{6.17}$$

Now, $|S| = S \cdot \text{sgn}(S)$, where

$$\text{sgn}(S) = \begin{cases} 1 & \text{if } S > 0, \\ 0 & \text{if } S = 0, \\ -1 & \text{if } S < 0. \end{cases}$$

Thus, from (6.17),

$$i \cdot \operatorname{sgn}(S) \cdot \mathcal{F}\left(\frac{\partial (\mathcal{R}f)(t, \theta)}{\partial t}\right)(S, \theta) = -|S| \, \mathcal{F}(\mathcal{R}f)(S, \theta). \tag{6.18}$$

It now follows from Theorem 6.2, the filtered back-projection formula, that

$$f(x, y) = \frac{-1}{2}\mathcal{B}\left\{\mathcal{F}^{-1}\left[i \cdot \operatorname{sgn}(S) \cdot \mathcal{F}\left(\frac{\partial (\mathcal{R}f)(t, \theta)}{\partial t}\right)(S, \theta)\right]\right\}(x, y). \tag{6.19}$$

That is quite a pile of symbols, so, historically, it has been simplified by defining a new transform, called the *Hilbert transform*, named for David Hilbert (1862–1943).

Definition 6.3. For a suitable function g defined on the real line, the *Hilbert transform* of g, denoted by $\mathcal{H}g$, is the function whose Fourier transform is equal to $i \cdot \operatorname{sgn} \cdot \mathcal{F}g$. That is, for each real number t, we define

$$\mathcal{H}g(t) = \mathcal{F}^{-1}\left[i \cdot \operatorname{sgn}(\omega) \cdot \mathcal{F}g(\omega)\right](t). \tag{6.20}$$

With this definition, (6.19) simplifies to the formula

$$f(x, y) = \frac{-1}{2}\mathcal{B}\left[\mathcal{H}\left(\frac{\partial (\mathcal{R}f)(t, \theta)}{\partial t}\right)(S, \theta)\right](x, y). \tag{6.21}$$

This is Radon's original inversion formula, though expressed here in contemporary notation. (See [43], or the English translation in [15].)

6.4 Exercises

1. Provide the logical explanation for each step in the proof of Theorem 6.1, the central slice theorem. (Note: The symbols $\mathcal{F}$ and $\mathcal{F}_2$ are used to denote the 1- and 2-dimensional Fourier transforms, respectively. The Radon transform is denoted by $\mathcal{R}$. In this problem, f is a function of 2-dimensional Cartesian coordinates, and $(S\cos(\theta), S\sin(\theta))$ is a typical point in 2-dimensional Cartesian space.)

$$\mathcal{F}_2 f(S\cos(\theta), S\sin(\theta)) = \int_{-\infty}^{\infty}\int_{-\infty}^{\infty} f(x, y)\, e^{-iS(x\cos(\theta)+y\sin(\theta))}\, dx\, dy \tag{6.22}$$

$$= \int_{-\infty}^{\infty}\int_{-\infty}^{\infty} f(t\cos(\theta) - s\sin(\theta),\ t\sin(\theta) + s\cos(\theta))\, e^{-iSt}\, ds\, dt \tag{6.23}$$

$$= \int_{-\infty}^{\infty} \left(\int_{-\infty}^{\infty} f(t\cos(\theta) - s\sin(\theta),\, t\sin(\theta) + s\cos(\theta))\, ds \right) e^{-iSt}\, dt \tag{6.24}$$

$$= \int_{-\infty}^{\infty} (\mathcal{R}f(t,\, \theta))\, e^{-iSt}\, dt \tag{6.25}$$

$$= \mathcal{F}(\mathcal{R}f)(S,\, \theta). \tag{6.26}$$

2. Provide a proof of the central slice theorem, Theorem 6.1, that reverses the order of the steps in the proof presented above. That is, start with the expression $\mathcal{F}(\mathcal{R}f)(S,\, \theta)$ and end with $\mathcal{F}_2 f(S\cos(\theta),\, S\sin(\theta))$.

3. Provide the logical explanation for each step in the derivation of Theorem 6.2, the filtered back-projection formula. (Note: The symbols $\mathcal{F}$ and $\mathcal{F}_2$ are used to denote the 1- and 2-dimensional Fourier transforms, respectively. The Radon transform is denoted by $\mathcal{R}$ and the back projection by $\mathcal{B}$. In this problem, f is a function of 2-dimensional Cartesian coordinates and $(x,\, y)$ is a typical point in the Cartesian plane.)

$$f(x,\, y) = \mathcal{F}_2^{-1} \mathcal{F}_2 f(x,\, y) \tag{6.27}$$

$$= \frac{1}{4\pi^2} \int_{-\infty}^{\infty} \int_{-\infty}^{\infty} \mathcal{F}_2 f(X,\, Y)\, e^{+i(xX+yY)}\, dX\, dY \tag{6.28}$$

$$= \frac{1}{4\pi^2} \int_{0}^{\pi} \int_{-\infty}^{\infty} \mathcal{F}_2 f(S\cos(\theta),\, S\sin(\theta))\, e^{+iS(x\cos(\theta)+y\sin(\theta))}\, |S|\, dS\, d\theta \tag{6.29}$$

$$= \frac{1}{4\pi^2} \int_{0}^{\pi} \int_{-\infty}^{\infty} \mathcal{F}(\mathcal{R}f)(S,\, \theta)\, e^{+iS(x\cos(\theta)+y\sin(\theta))}\, |S|\, dS\, d\theta \tag{6.30}$$

$$= \frac{1}{2\pi} \int_{0}^{\pi} \mathcal{F}^{-1}\left[|S|\, \mathcal{F}(\mathcal{R}f)(S,\, \theta)\right](x\cos(\theta) + y\sin(\theta),\, \theta)\, d\theta \tag{6.31}$$

$$= \frac{1}{2} \mathcal{B}\left\{ \mathcal{F}^{-1}\left[|S|\, \mathcal{F}(\mathcal{R}f)(S,\, \theta)\right] \right\}(x,\, y). \tag{6.32}$$

7

Filters and Convolution

7.1 Introduction

Of constant concern in the analysis of signals is the presence of *noise*, a term which here means more or less any effect that corrupts a signal. This corruption may arise from background radiation, stray signals that interfere with the main signal, errors in the measurement of the actual signal, or what have you. In order to remove the effects of noise and form a clearer picture of the actual signal, a *filter* is applied.

For a first example of a filter, consider that the noise present in a signal is often *random*. That means that the *average* amount of noise over time should be 0. Consider also that noise often has a high frequency, so the graph of the noise signal is fuzzy and jaggedy. That means that the amount of noise should average out to 0 over a fairly short time interval. So, let $T > 0$ be a positive real number and let f represent a noisy signal. For each fixed value of x, the average value of f over the interval $x - T \le t \le x + T$ is given by

$$f_{\text{ave}}(x) = \frac{1}{2T} \int_{t=x-T}^{x+T} f(t)\, dt. \tag{7.1}$$

The function f_{ave} that has just been defined represents a *filtered* version of the original signal f. For an appropriate value of T, the noise should average out to 0 over the interval, so f_{ave} would be close to the noise-free signal that we are trying to recover. If the value of T is too large, then some interesting features of the true signal may get smoothed out too much. If the choice of T is too small, then the time interval may be too short for the randomized noise to average out to 0.

Electronic supplementary material The online version of this chapter (doi: 10.1007/978-3-319-22665-1_7) contains supplementary material, which is available to authorized users.

© Springer International Publishing Switzerland 2015
T.G. Feeman, *The Mathematics of Medical Imaging*, Springer Undergraduate
Texts in Mathematics and Technology, DOI 10.1007/978-3-319-22665-1_7

A deeper analysis of (7.1) suggests that we consider the function $\phi = \Pi_T/(2T)$, where

$$\Pi_T(t) = \begin{cases} 1 & \text{if } -T \le t \le T, \\ 0 & \text{if } |t| > T. \end{cases} \tag{7.2}$$

Notice that

$$\int_{-\infty}^{\infty} \phi(t)\, dt = \frac{1}{2T} \cdot \int_{-T}^{T} \Pi_T(t)\, dt = 1.$$

Also, for each fixed value of x, we get

$$\phi(x-t) = \begin{cases} \frac{1}{2T} & \text{if } x - T \le t \le x + T, \\ 0 & \text{otherwise.} \end{cases} \tag{7.3}$$

Hence, for any given function f and any fixed value of x, we get

$$f(t)\,\phi(x-t) = \begin{cases} \frac{1}{2T} f(t) & \text{if } x - T \le t \le x + T, \\ 0 & \text{otherwise,} \end{cases} \tag{7.4}$$

from which it follows that the integral in (7.1) is the same as the integral

$$f_{\text{ave}}(x) = \int_{t=-\infty}^{\infty} f(t)\,\phi(x-t)\, dt. \tag{7.5}$$

Computationally, the function f_{ave} represents a moving average of the value of f over intervals of width $2T$. This technique is used for the analysis of all sorts of signals — radio, electrical, microwave, audio — and also for things we might not think of as being signals, like long-term behavior of stock market prices.

Graphically, the graph of $\phi(x-t)$ as a function of t is obtained by flipping the graph of ϕ over from right to left and then sliding this flipped graph along the t-axis until it is centered at x instead of at 0. This reflected-and-translated version of ϕ is then superimposed on the graph of f, and the area under the graph of the resulting product is computed. To generate the graph of f_{ave}, we reflect the graph of ϕ and then slide the reflected graph across the graph of f, stopping at each x value to compute the area underneath the product where the graphs overlap.

Example 7.1. Consider a simple square wave:

$$f(t) = \Pi_a(t) = \begin{cases} 1 \text{ if } |t| \le a, \\ 0 \text{ if } |t| > a. \end{cases}$$

Take $\phi = \Pi_T/(2T)$ as above. Let's also assume that $a \ge T$.

For any given value of x, the product $f(t) \cdot \phi(x-t)$ will vanish at values of t outside the intersection of the intervals $x - T \le t \le x + T$ and $-a \le t \le a$. The value of the integral $\int_{t=-\infty}^{\infty} f(t) \cdot \phi(x-t)\, dt$ will be equal to the length of this overlap multiplied by $1/(2T)$.

There are three sets of values of x to consider. First, if $|x| > T + a$, then it is impossible to have *both* $|t| \le a$ *and* $|x - t| \le T$. So $f(t) \cdot \phi(x - t) = 0$ for all t in this case. Next, for x satisfying $|x| \le a - T$, we have both $-a \le x - T$ and $x + T \le a$. Hence, $f(t) \cdot \phi(x - t) = 1/(2T)$ whenever $x - T \le t \le x + T$; therefore,

$$\int_{t=-\infty}^{\infty} f(t) \cdot \phi(x - t)\, dt = \int_{t=x-T}^{x+T} \left(\frac{1}{2T}\right) dt = 1 \, .$$

Finally, consider x such that $a - T \le |x| \le a + T$. In this case, the intersection of the intervals $[x - T, x + T]$ and $[-a, a]$ is either the interval $[x - T, a]$ or the interval $[-a, x + T]$, depending on whether x is positive or negative, respectively. In either event, this intersection is an interval of width $a + T - |x|$. Hence, for such x, we get

$$\int_{t=-\infty}^{\infty} f(t) \cdot \phi(x - t)\, dt = \frac{1}{2T} \cdot (a + T - |x|) \, .$$

Combining these cases, we have shown that the filtered function f_{ave}, as in (7.5), is given by

$$f_{\mathrm{ave}}(x) = \begin{cases} 1 & \text{if } |x| \le a - T, \\ \frac{1}{2T} \cdot (a + T - |x|) & \text{if } a - T \le |x| \le a + T, \\ 0 & \text{if } |x| > a + T. \end{cases} \tag{7.6}$$

Figure 7.1 shows an example of this. We see that, where the graph of f is a box (square wave) on the interval $[-a, a]$, the graph of f_{ave} has been spread out over the interval $[-a - T, a + T]$. The sides of the graph of f_{ave} are no longer vertical but sloped, with slopes

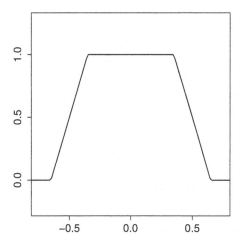

Fig. 7.1. The convolution of two boxes, in this case $\sqcap_{0.5}$ and $\sqcap_{0.15}$, has the shape of a truncated tent. (If the boxes have the same width, then the convolution will be a tent.)

$\pm 1/(2T)$. Instead of a signal that starts and ends abruptly, as with the box, the smoothed-out signal fades in and fades out more gradually. In the case where $a = T$, the box actually becomes a tent. Perhaps we can visualize filling a rectangular box with dry sand. When the box is turned upside down and lifted away, the pile of sand will lose its box shape as the edges collapse. In the extreme case, the pile of sand will collapse into a cone.

7.2 Convolution

When some other function g is used in place of $\sqcap_T/(2T)$ in the integral in (7.5), then the resulting function is not a simple moving average of the value of f over successive intervals. But we do get a modified version of f that has been "filtered" in a way that is determined by the function g. We make the following formal definition.

Definition 7.2. Given two functions f and g (defined and integrable on the real line), the *convolution* of f and g is denoted by $f * g$ and defined by

$$(f * g)(x) := \int_{t=-\infty}^{\infty} f(t)\, g(x - t)\, dt \ \text{ for } x \in \mathbb{R}. \tag{7.7}$$

For instance, the function f_{ave} in (7.5) is the same as the convolution $f * \phi$, where $\phi = \sqcap_T/(2T)$. Graphically, the graph of $f * g$ can be obtained by reflecting the graph of g across the y-axis, then sliding the reflected graph across the graph of f, stopping at each x to compute the integral of the product where the two graphs overlap.

Example 7.3. The formula for the convolution $\sqcap_a * (\sqcap_T/(2T))$ is given in (7.6).

Example 7.4. For the tent function $\bigwedge(t) = \begin{cases} 1 - |t| & \text{if } -1 \le t \le 1, \\ 0 & \text{if } |t| > 1, \end{cases}$ the convolution $\bigwedge * \bigwedge$ is piecewise cubic on the interval $-2 \le x \le 2$ and vanishes outside that interval.

In general, it is not so easy to compute the convolution of two functions by hand. The most manageable situation occurs if one of the functions is a box function $k \cdot \sqcap_T$. Another helpful observation is that, if f vanishes outside the interval $[a, b]$ and g vanishes outside the interval $[c, d]$, then the convolution $f * g$ vanishes outside the interval $[a + c, b + d]$. The proof of this is left as an exercise.

7.2.1 Some properties of convolution

Commutativity. For suitable functions f and g, we get

$$f * g = g * f.$$

Proof. For each real number x, by definition

$$(f * g)(x) = \int_{t=-\infty}^{\infty} f(t)\, g(x-t)\, dt.$$

Make a change of variables with $u = x - t$. Then $du = -dt$ and $t = (x - u)$. Also, when $t = -\infty$, then $u = \infty$ and, when $t = \infty$, then $u = -\infty$. (Remember that x is fixed throughout this process). Thus, the previous integral becomes

$$\int_{u=\infty}^{-\infty} f(x-u)\, g(u)\, (-du)$$

which is the same as the integral

$$\int_{u=-\infty}^{\infty} g(u) f(x-u)\, du.$$

This last integral is exactly the definition of $(g * f)(x)$. Thus, $f * g = g * f$ as claimed. □

Linearity. For suitable functions f, g_1, and g_2, and for scalars α and β, we get

$$f * (\alpha g_1 + \beta g_2) = \alpha(f * g_1) + \beta(f * g_2).$$

This property follows immediately from the fact that integration is linear. Combining this with the commutativity result, we also get that

$$(\alpha g_1 + \beta g_2) * f = \alpha(g_1 * f) + \beta(g_2 * f).$$

Shifting. Given a function f and a real number a, let f_a denote the shifted (translated) function

$$f_a(x) = f(x-a).$$

Then, for suitable g, we get

$$\begin{aligned}
(g * f_a)(x) &= \int_{t=-\infty}^{\infty} g(t) f_a(x-t)\, dt \\
&= \int_{t=-\infty}^{\infty} g(t) f(x-t-a)\, dt \\
&= \int_{t=-\infty}^{\infty} g(t) f((x-a)-t)\, dt \\
&= (g * f)(x-a) \\
&= (g * f)_a(x).
\end{aligned}$$

Similarly,

$$(g_a * f)(x) = \int_{t=-\infty}^{\infty} g_a(t) f(x-t) \, dt$$

$$= \int_{t=-\infty}^{\infty} g(t-a) f(x-t) \, dt$$

$$= \int_{t=-\infty}^{\infty} g(t-a) f((x-a)-(t-a)) \, dt$$

$$= \int_{s=-\infty}^{\infty} g(s) f((x-a)-s) \, ds \quad \text{where } s = t-a$$

$$= (g * f)(x-a)$$

$$= (g * f)_a(x) \, .$$

Convolution with δ. The convolution of an arbitrary function with the Dirac delta function yields an interesting result — it isolates the value of the function at a specific point. Specifically, for each real number x, compute

$$(f * \delta)(x) = \int_{t=-\infty}^{\infty} f(t) \, \delta(x-t) \, dt = f(x) \, ,$$

where we have used the facts that $\delta(x-t) = 0$ unless $t = x$ and that $\int_{-\infty}^{\infty} \delta(s) \, ds = 1$. In other words, convolution with δ acts like the identity map:

$$(f * \delta)(x) = f(x) \text{ for all } x; \ f * \delta = f \, . \tag{7.8}$$

7.3 Filter resolution

The convolution of a function f with the δ function reproduces f exactly; so this filter has perfect resolution. More generally, let ϕ be a nonnegative function with a single maximum value M attained at $x = 0$. Suppose also that ϕ is increasing for $x < 0$ and decreasing for $x > 0$. (For example, ϕ could be a Gaussian or a tent.) Let the numbers x_1 and x_2 satisfy $x_1 < 0 < x_2$ and $\phi(x_1) = \phi(x_2) = M/2$, half the maximum value of ϕ. The distance $(x_2 - x_1)$ is called the *full width half maximum* of the function ϕ, denoted FWHM(ϕ). For the filter of convolution with ϕ, the resolution of the filter is *defined* to be equal to FWHM(ϕ).

The idea is that a function ϕ having a smaller FWHM is pointier or spikier than a function with a larger FWHM and, hence, looks more like the δ function. So the resolution is better if the filter function ϕ has a smaller FWHM.

Here is a graphical way to see how the resolution of a filter is related to the FWHM of the filter function. Suppose a signal S consists of two impulses, two instantaneous blips, separated by a positive distance of a. Using the graphical approach to convolution, where we slide the reflected graph of the filter function ϕ across the graph of S, we see that, if $a > \text{FWHM}(\phi)$, then the sliding copy of ϕ will slide past the first impulse before it really reaches the second one. Hence, the graph of $(\phi * S)$ will have two distinct peaks, like S. But if a is less than $\text{FWHM}(\phi)$, then the sliding copy of ϕ will overlap both impulses at once, so the two peaks will start to blend together. The detail in the original signal is getting blurry. For a sufficiently small, the graph of $(\phi * S)$ will have only one peak, so the detail in S will have been lost completely. Overall, we see that the smallest distance between distinct features (the spikes) in the signal S that will still be distinct in the filtered signal $(\phi * S)$ is $a = \text{FWHM}(\phi)$.

For a computational perspective, take $a > 0$ and let S be the signal $S(x) = \delta(x) + \delta(x-a)$. Suppose also that the filter function ϕ is symmetric about $x = 0$ and achieves its maximum value M there. Thus, ϕ attains its half-maximum $M/2$ when $x = \pm(1/2)\cdot\text{FWHM}(\phi)$. Let's also assume that the graph of ϕ tapers off fairly quickly away from 0, meaning that $\phi(x) \approx 0$ when $|x| \geq \text{FWHM}(\phi)$. With this setup, the convolution is $\phi*S(x) = \phi(x)+\phi(x-a)$, the sum of two copies of ϕ, one of which has been shifted to the right by a units. (Here we have used the shifting property of convolution together with formula (7.8) above.) So what happens if $a = \text{FWHM}(\phi)$? Well, then we get $\phi * S(a/2) = \phi(a/2) + \phi(-a/2) = M/2 + M/2 = M$. We also get $\phi * S(0) = M + \phi(-a)$ and $\phi * S(a) = \phi(a) + M$, both of which are close to M in value, given our assumptions about the graph of ϕ. In other words, with $a = \text{FWHM}(\phi)$, the filtered signal $(\phi * S)$ will be near M in value on the entire interval $0 \leq x \leq a$. The two distinct spikes in S will get smeared or blurred across an interval. If $a < \text{FWHM}(\phi)$, the blurring gets even worse. The detail in the signal has been lost! On the other hand, suppose $a = 2 \cdot \text{FWHM}(\phi)$. Then ϕ will achieve its half-maximum value of $M/2$ at $\pm a/4$. So $\phi * S(0) = \phi(0) + \phi(-a) \approx M$ and $\phi * S(a) = \phi(a) + \phi(0) \approx M$. The filtered signal will have two distinct peaks, at or near $x = 0$ and $x = a$, with a valley in between, at $x = a/2$. The original detail has been preserved.

Thus, the choice of the filter function has a direct effect on the resolution of the filtered signal.

Example 7.5. FWHM of a box. The box function

$$\sqcap_T(x) = \begin{cases} 1 \text{ if } |x| \leq T, \\ 0 \text{ if } |x| > T, \end{cases}$$

doesn't satisfy the condition specified above that the filter should attain its maximum at a single point. Nonetheless, these functions make good filters in applications. So we'll cheat and declare the FWHM of a box to be the width of the box; that is, $\text{FWHM}(\sqcap_T) = 2T$.

Example 7.6. FWHM of a tent. For $T > 0$, take

$$\phi_T(x) = \begin{cases} \frac{1}{T}(T - |x|) & \text{if } |x| \leq T, \\ 0 & \text{if } |x| > T. \end{cases}$$

The graph of ϕ is a tent with a maximum height of $M = 1$, attained at $x = 0$. Since $\phi(\pm T/2) = 1/2$, it follows that $\text{FWHM}(\phi) = T$.

Example 7.7. FWHM of a Gaussian. For ω real, let $F(\omega) = e^{-B\omega^2}$, where B is a positive constant. The maximum value of F is $F(0) = 1$. Thus, half maximum is achieved when $e^{-B\omega^2} = 1/2$, or when $\omega = \pm\sqrt{\ln(2)/B}$. Therefore,

$$\text{FWHM} = 2\sqrt{\ln(2)/B}$$

for this function.

Example 7.8. FWHM of a Lorentzian. A signal of the form

$$g(\omega) = \frac{T_2}{1 + 4\pi^2 T_2^2(\omega - \omega_0)^2},$$

where T_2 is a positive constant and the signal is centered around the angular frequency ω_0, is called a *Lorentzian*. These signals are important in magnetic resonance imaging (MRI), in which context the constant T_2 is one of the so-called *relaxation constants*. We leave it as an exercise to show that the FWHM of this Lorentzian is $1/(\pi T_2)$.

7.4 Convolution and the Fourier transform

For suitable functions f and g, the product of their respective Fourier transforms, evaluated at ω, is

$$\mathcal{F}f(\omega) \cdot \mathcal{F}g(\omega) = \int_{x=-\infty}^{\infty} f(x)\, e^{-i\omega x}\, dx \cdot \int_{y=-\infty}^{\infty} g(y)\, e^{-i\omega y}\, dy. \tag{7.9}$$

Keep in mind that x and y are just "dummy" variables here. Now, introduce a new variable s such that, for each fixed value of x, we have $y = s - x$. Thus $dy = ds$, and hence the right-hand side of (7.9) becomes

$$\int_{x=-\infty}^{\infty} f(x)\, e^{-i\omega x}\, dx \cdot \int_{s=-\infty}^{\infty} g(s - x)\, e^{-i\omega(s-x)}\, ds. \tag{7.10}$$

The first integral in (7.10) is independent of s, so we may move it inside the other integral. Since $e^{-i\omega x} \cdot e^{-i\omega(s-x)} = e^{-i\omega s}$, this yields

$$\int_{s=-\infty}^{\infty} \left(\int_{x=-\infty}^{\infty} f(x)\, g(s-x)\, dx \right) e^{-i\omega s}\, ds. \tag{7.11}$$

Notice now that the inner integral in (7.11) is exactly $(f * g)(s)$, while the outer integral is the Fourier transform of the inner integral, evaluated at ω. That is, (7.11) is the same as

$$\int_{s=-\infty}^{\infty} (f * g)(s)\, e^{-i\omega s}\, ds = \mathcal{F}(f * g)(\omega). \tag{7.12}$$

Thus, we have established the following property.

Theorem 7.9. *For suitable functions f and g,*

$$\mathcal{F}f \cdot \mathcal{F}g = \mathcal{F}(f * g). \tag{7.13}$$

So, we see that the Fourier transform of a convolution is just the product of the individual transforms. This relationship will play a significant role in what is to come. We might wonder as well what happens if we apply the Fourier transform to a product. The result is almost as clean as in the previous theorem, except for a factor of $1/2\pi$ that creeps in.

Theorem 7.10. *For suitable functions f and g,*

$$\mathcal{F}(f \cdot g) = \frac{1}{2\pi}\, (\mathcal{F}f) * (\mathcal{F}g). \tag{7.14}$$

Proof. Given f and g, for simplicity denote $\mathcal{F}f$ and $\mathcal{F}g$ by F and G, respectively. The Fourier transform of the product $f \cdot g$, evaluated at an arbitrary real number ω, is

$$\mathcal{F}(f \cdot g)(\omega)$$

$$= \int_{x=-\infty}^{\infty} f(x) g(x)\, e^{-i\omega x}\, dx$$

$$= \frac{1}{4\pi^2} \cdot \int_{x=-\infty}^{\infty} \left(\int_{\nu=-\infty}^{\infty} F(\nu) e^{+i\nu x}\, d\nu \right) \left(\int_{\zeta=-\infty}^{\infty} G(\zeta) e^{+i\zeta x}\, d\zeta \right) e^{-i\omega x}\, dx$$

$$= \frac{1}{4\pi^2} \cdot \int_{\nu=-\infty}^{\infty} F(\nu) \left(\int_{\zeta=-\infty}^{\infty} G(\zeta) \left(\int_{x=-\infty}^{\infty} e^{+i(\nu+\zeta-\omega)x}\, dx \right) d\zeta \right) d\nu.$$

Observe that the inner integral, $\int_{x=-\infty}^{\infty} e^{+i(\nu+\zeta-\omega)x}\, dx$, represents (2π) times the inverse Fourier transform of the constant function 1 evaluated at $(\nu + \zeta - \omega)$. But $\mathcal{F}^{-1}(1) = \delta$, so,

$$\int_{x=-\infty}^{\infty} e^{+i(\nu+\zeta-\omega)x}\, dx = (2\pi) \cdot \delta(\nu + \zeta - \omega).$$

Moreover, $\delta(v + \zeta - \omega) = 0$ except when $\zeta = \omega - v$. Hence, from (5.13),

$$\int_{\zeta=-\infty}^{\infty} G(\zeta) \left(\int_{x=-\infty}^{\infty} e^{+i(v+\zeta-\omega)x}\, dx \right) d\zeta$$

$$= 2\pi \int_{\zeta=-\infty}^{\infty} G(\zeta)\, \delta(v + \zeta - \omega)\, d\zeta = 2\pi\, G(\omega - v).$$

Continuing from where we left off, we now see that

$$\mathcal{F}(f \cdot g)(\omega)$$

$$= \frac{1}{4\pi^2} \cdot \int_{v=-\infty}^{\infty} F(v) \left(\int_{\zeta=-\infty}^{\infty} G(\zeta) \left(\int_{x=-\infty}^{\infty} e^{+i(v+\zeta-\omega)x}\, dx \right) d\zeta \right) dv$$

$$= \frac{1}{2\pi} \cdot \int_{v=-\infty}^{\infty} F(v)\, G(\omega - v)\, dv$$

$$= \frac{1}{2\pi} \cdot (F * G)(\omega),$$

which establishes the claim. □

7.5   The Rayleigh–Plancherel theorem

Theorem 7.11. Rayleigh–Plancherel. *Let f be an integrable function. If either the function f or its Fourier transform $\mathcal{F}f$ is square-integrable on the real line, then so is the other and*

$$\int_{-\infty}^{\infty} |f(x)|^2\, dx = \frac{1}{2\pi} \int_{-\infty}^{\infty} |\mathcal{F}f(\omega)|^2\, d\omega. \tag{7.15}$$

Before looking at a proof of this statement, note that both integrands are nonnegative functions even if f or $\mathcal{F}f$ has complex number values. The function $|\mathcal{F}f(\omega)|^2$ is called the *power spectrum* of f, and in some physical applications actually does represent the total power (measured in watts, for example) of a signal at a given frequency. In the same sort of setting, the integral on the right in (7.15) represents a measure of the total amount of power present in the system.

Computationally, the value of the theorem is that one of the integrals might be comparatively easy to evaluate while the other, on its own, may be difficult.

Example 7.12. Take

$$f(x) = \begin{cases} 1 & \text{if } -1 \leq x \leq 1, \\ 0 & \text{if } |x| > 1. \end{cases}$$

Then

$$\int_{-\infty}^{\infty} |f(x)|^2 \, dx = \int_{-1}^{1} 1 \, dx = 2.$$

We have seen before that $\mathcal{F}f(\omega) = 2\dfrac{\sin(\omega)}{\omega}$. Hence, by (7.15),

$$\int_{-\infty}^{\infty} \frac{\sin^2(\omega)}{\omega^2} \, d\omega = \pi \, .$$

Rayleigh established this result in 1889 and used it in his analysis of blackbody radiation. Where Rayleigh tacitly assumed that both integrals would be finite, Plancherel proved, in 1910, that the existence of one or the other integral is indeed the only hypothesis required. In other words, the relation (7.15) holds whenever either integral exists.

Now for the proof.

Proof of Theorem 7.11. Let f be an integrable function and suppose that either f or $\mathcal{F}f$ is square-integrable. We have

$$\int_{-\infty}^{\infty} |f(x)|^2 \, dx = \int_{-\infty}^{\infty} f(x)\overline{f(x)} \, dx$$

$$= \int_{-\infty}^{\infty} f(x)\overline{f(x)} \, e^{-i(0)x} \, dx$$

$$= \mathcal{F}(f \cdot \bar{f})(0)$$

$$= \frac{1}{2\pi} \left[(\mathcal{F}f) * (\mathcal{F}\bar{f}) \right](0) \text{ by (7.14)}$$

$$= \frac{1}{2\pi} \int_{-\infty}^{\infty} \mathcal{F}f(\omega) \, \mathcal{F}\bar{f}(0 - \omega) \, d\omega$$

$$= \frac{1}{2\pi} \int_{-\infty}^{\infty} \mathcal{F}f(\omega) \, \overline{\mathcal{F}f(\omega)} \, d\omega \text{ by (5.10)}$$

$$= \frac{1}{2\pi} \int_{-\infty}^{\infty} |\mathcal{F}f(\omega)|^2 \, d\omega.$$

Hence, provided one of these integrals is finite, then so is the other and the desired relation holds. □

7.6 Convolution in 2-dimensional space

For two functions whose inputs are polar coordinates in the plane, the convolution is defined in terms of the radial variable only. That is, for $f(t, \theta)$ and $g(t, \theta)$, we define

$$(f * g)(t, \theta) = \int_{s=-\infty}^{\infty} f(s, \theta) \cdot g(t - s, \theta) \, ds. \tag{7.16}$$

For two functions whose inputs are Cartesian coordinates in the plane, the convolution incorporates both variables. That is, for $F(x, y)$ and $G(x, y)$, we define

$$(F * G)(x, y) = \int_{t=-\infty}^{\infty} \int_{s=-\infty}^{\infty} F(s, t) \cdot G(x - s, y - t) \, ds \, dt. \tag{7.17}$$

As in one dimension, convolution is *commutative*: $f * g = g * f$ and $F * G = G * F$.

7.7 Convolution, $\mathcal{B}$, $\mathcal{R}$, and δ

Given functions $g(t, \theta)$ (in polar coordinates) and $f(x, y)$ (in Cartesian coordinates), recall that the back projection and Radon transform are defined by

$$\mathcal{B}g(x, y) = \frac{1}{\pi} \int_{\theta=0}^{\pi} g(x \cos(\theta) + y \sin(\theta), \theta) \, d\theta \tag{7.18}$$

and

$$\mathcal{R}f(t, \theta) = \int_{s=-\infty}^{\infty} f(t \cos(\theta) - s \sin(\theta), t \sin(\theta) + s \cos(\theta)) \, ds. \tag{7.19}$$

Proposition 7.13. *(See [39], Theorem 1.3) For suitable functions $g(t, \theta)$ and $f(x, y)$, and arbitrary real numbers X and Y, we have*

$$(\mathcal{B}g * f)(X, Y) = \mathcal{B}(g * \mathcal{R}f)(X, Y). \tag{7.20}$$

Proof. From (7.17) and (7.18), we compute

$$(\mathcal{B}g * f)(X, Y) = \int_{-\infty}^{\infty} \int_{-\infty}^{\infty} \mathcal{B}g(X - x, Y - y) \cdot f(x, y) \, dx \, dy$$

$$= \frac{1}{\pi} \int_{-\infty}^{\infty} \int_{-\infty}^{\infty} \left[\int_{0}^{\pi} g((X - x) \cos(\theta) + (Y - y) \sin(\theta), \theta) d\theta \right] f(x, y) dx dy.$$

Now substitute $x = t \cos(\theta) - s \sin(\theta)$ and $y = t \sin(\theta) + s \cos(\theta)$. Keeping in mind that $ds \, dt = dx \, dy$ and using (7.19), the preceding integral becomes

$$= \frac{1}{\pi} \int_{0}^{\pi} \int_{-\infty}^{\infty} g(X \cos(\theta) + Y \sin(\theta) - t, \theta) \cdot \mathcal{R}f(t, \theta) \, dt \, d\theta$$

$$= \frac{1}{\pi} \int_0^\pi (g * \mathcal{R}f)(X\cos(\theta) + Y\sin(\theta), \theta)\, d\theta \quad \text{by (7.16)}$$

$$= \mathcal{B}(g * \mathcal{R}f)(X, Y) \quad \text{by (7.18).}$$

This proves the claim. $\qquad\qquad\qquad\qquad\qquad\qquad\qquad\qquad\qquad\qquad\qquad\qquad\quad$ □

We observed earlier that applying the back projection to the Radon transform of an attenuation function resulted in a smoothing out of the attenuation function. We can now use Proposition 7.13 to make this more concrete. Indeed, suppose we take g, in (7.20), to be the 2-dimensional Dirac δ function. Since $\delta * \mathcal{R}f = \mathcal{R}f$, the right-hand side of the conclusion is just $\mathcal{B}(\mathcal{R}f)$, while the left-hand side is $\mathcal{B}\delta * f$. Thus, when we apply the back projection to the Radon transform of a function, the effect is to smooth the function by taking its convolution with the filter $\mathcal{B}\delta$. So now, of course, we're curious to know what the back projection of the δ function is!

To find the answer, look at the limit formulation in (5.32), and, for convenience, set

$$h_a(r, \theta) = \begin{cases} \frac{1}{2a} & \text{if } -a \le r \le a, \\ 0 & \text{if } |r| > a. \end{cases}$$

For each point (x, y) in the plane and each value of θ, we know that the line $\ell_{x\cos(\theta)+y\sin(\theta),\theta}$ passes through (x, y). So, given a small positive value of a, we are interested in those values of θ for which $|x\cos(\theta) + y\sin(\theta)| \le a$. In Figure 7.2, we see that the angle labeled α satisfies $\sin(\alpha) = a/\sqrt{x^2 + y^2}$. Since a is small, the angle α is also small and, so, $\alpha \approx \sin(\alpha)$. It follows that the interval of values of θ that we want will have width $2\alpha \approx 2a/\sqrt{x^2 + y^2}$.

Thus,

$$\mathcal{B}h_a(x, y) = \frac{1}{\pi} \int_0^\pi h_a(x\cos(\theta) + y\sin(\theta), \theta)\, d\theta$$

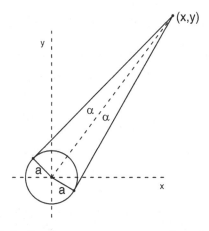

Fig. 7.2. The set of θ for which the line $\ell_{x\cos(\theta)+y\sin(\theta),\theta}$ passes through (x, y) has width 2α.

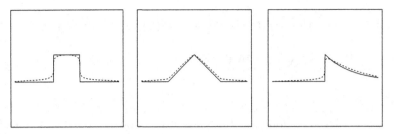

Fig. 7.3. Each figure shows cross sections of the graph of an attenuation-coefficient function (solid line) with the back projection of its Radon transform (dashed line).

$$\approx \frac{1}{\pi} \cdot \left(\frac{1}{2a} \right) \cdot \frac{2a}{\sqrt{x^2 + y^2}}$$

$$= \frac{1}{\pi \sqrt{x^2 + y^2}} \cdot$$

Letting $a \to 0^+$ improves the approximations involved, so we conclude that

$$\mathcal{B}\delta(x, y) = \frac{1}{\pi \sqrt{x^2 + y^2}} . \tag{7.21}$$

Here is what we have now shown.

Corollary 7.14. *For a suitable attenuation-coefficient function f,*

$$\mathcal{B}(\mathcal{R}f) = \frac{1}{\pi} \left(\frac{1}{\sqrt{x^2 + y^2}} \right) * f . \tag{7.22}$$

Example with R 7.15. Figure 7.3 shows cross sections for several pairings of an attenuation-coefficient function with the back projection of its Radon transform. The back projections were computed as the convolution in (7.22). The smoothing effect is the same as what we saw before, only now we have a precise way to quantify it.

The `convolve` procedure in R implements a discrete version of convolution that we will discuss in Chapter 8. Moreover, this procedure does not "flip over" the second operand and, so, computes the so-called cross correlation of two (discretized) functions. To get true convolution, we need to reverse the list of values of the second function. Also, the value of $\mathcal{B}\delta$ has been modified slightly in the following example to avoid evaluation at 0.

```
#B(Rf) computed as convolution B(delta)*f
xval=(.01)*(-200:200)#list of x-coord
f1=1*(abs(xval)<=0.5)#vals of f1
Bdelta=1/(pi*abs(xval+.0025))#vals of B(delta)
f1.new=convolve(f1,rev(Bdelta),type="open")
plot(c(-2,2),c(0,1),type = "n",asp=1,xlab="",ylab="")
```

```
lines(xval,fval,lwd=2)
lines(xval,f.new[201:601]/max(f.new[201:601]),lwd=2,lty=2)
## other functions
f2=(1-abs(xval))*(abs(xval)<=1)
f2.new=convolve(f2,rev(Bdelta),type="open")
f3=exp(-1*xval)*(xval>=0)
f3.new=convolve(f3,rev(Bdelta),type="open")
```

7.8   Low-pass filters

Let us return our attention to the filtered back-projection formula,

$$f(x, y) = \frac{1}{2}\mathcal{B}\left\{\mathcal{F}^{-1}\left[|S|\,\mathcal{F}\,(\mathcal{R}f\,)\,(S,\,\theta)\right]\right\}(x,\,y)\,, \tag{7.23}$$

where f is some suitable function defined in the xy-plane.

Suppose there were a function $\phi(t)$ whose Fourier transform satisfied $\mathcal{F}\phi(S) = |S|$. That is, suppose $\mathcal{F}\phi$ were equal to the absolute-value function. Then we would get

$$|S|\,\mathcal{F}\,(\mathcal{R}f\,)\,(S,\,\theta) = [\mathcal{F}\phi \cdot \mathcal{F}\,(\mathcal{R}f\,)]\,(S,\,\theta).$$

This is the product of two Fourier transforms, which we now know is equal to the Fourier transform of the convolution of the two functions. So we would have

$$|S|\,\mathcal{F}\,(\mathcal{R}f\,)\,(S,\,\theta) = \mathcal{F}\,(\phi * \mathcal{R}f\,)\,(S,\,\theta).$$

Hence, we would have

$$\mathcal{F}^{-1}\left[|S|\,\mathcal{F}\,(\mathcal{R}f\,)\,(S,\,\theta)\right] = \mathcal{F}^{-1}\left[\mathcal{F}\,(\phi * \mathcal{R}f\,)\,(S,\,\theta)\right]$$
$$= (\phi * \mathcal{R}f\,)\,(t,\,\theta).$$

Substituting this into (7.23), we would get

$$f(x,\,y) = \frac{1}{2}\mathcal{B}\,(\phi * \mathcal{R}f\,)\,(x,\,y). \tag{7.24}$$

Thus, reconstruction of f would require the convolution, or filtering, of $\mathcal{R}f$, the data from the X-ray machine, with ϕ followed by an application of the back projection to that. That doesn't sound so terrible, *except that there is no such function ϕ. The absolute-value function is not the Fourier transform of any function.*

So we might as well ignore all of the preceding discussion, right? Well, not so fast. The filtered back-projection formula (7.23) gives a recipe for reconstructing f, but in practice the recipe has a problem. The function $|S| \, \mathcal{F} \, (\mathcal{R}f) \, (S, \, \theta)$ in the formula is highly sensitive to noise. The value of S represents a frequency that is present in a signal. So, if the Radon transform $\mathcal{R}f$, representing the X-ray data, has a component at a high frequency, then that component is magnified by the factor $|S|$. That means that noise present in the data gets exaggerated, an effect which corrupts the reconstructed image. Thus, in practice, we don't really want to use the factor $|S|$ anyway.

In place of $|S|$, we use a function that is close to the absolute-value function for S near 0 but that vanishes when the value of $|S|$ is large. Such a function is called a *low-pass filter* because the lower frequencies are not affected by its presence while higher frequencies, including noise, get cut off. Also, in order to use the modification (7.24) of the filtered back-projection formula, we want the function that replaces $|S|$ to be the Fourier transform of something. That is, we want to replace $|S|$ with a function of the form $A = \mathcal{F}\phi$, where A is nonzero on some finite interval and zero outside that interval.

Definition 7.16. A function ϕ whose Fourier transform is nonzero on some finite interval and zero outside that interval is called a *band-limited function*.

So, using this terminology, we want to replace $|S|$ in the filtered back-projection formula by a low-pass filter that is the Fourier transform of a band-limited function. The price of doing this is that *the formula (7.24) is no longer exact*, but gives only an approximation for f:

$$f(x, y) \approx \frac{1}{2} \mathcal{B} \left(\mathcal{F}^{-1}A * \mathcal{R}f \right) (x, y). \tag{7.25}$$

To design a low-pass filter to replace the absolute-value function, we typically use a function of the form

$$A(\omega) = |\omega| \cdot F(\omega) \cdot \sqcap_L(\omega) , \tag{7.26}$$

for some number $L > 0$. Thus, $A(\omega)$ vanishes for $|\omega| > L$ and has the value $|\omega| \cdot F(\omega)$ when $|\omega| \leq L$. Near the origin, the value of A should be close to the absolute value, so we want F to be an even function for which $F(0) = 1$. Also, choosing A to be an even function guarantees that $\phi = \mathcal{F}^{-1}A$ is real-valued. In general, the function $F \cdot \sqcap_L$, by which $| \cdot |$ is multiplied, is called the *window function*.

Example 7.17. Low-pass filters. Here are some of the low-pass filters most commonly used in medical imaging. We will analyze them more closely in Section 8.3. Their graphs are shown in Figure 7.4.

- The *Ram–Lak filter*:

$$A_1(\omega) = |\omega| \cdot \sqcap_L(\omega) = \begin{cases} |\omega| \text{ if } |\omega| \leq L, \\ 0 \ \text{ if } |\omega| > L, \end{cases} \tag{7.27}$$

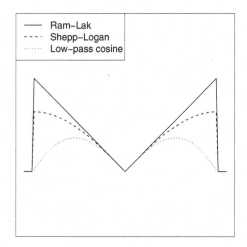

Fig. 7.4. The graphs of three popular low-pass filters are shown.

where $L > 0$. This is simply a truncation of the absolute-value function to a finite interval. It is the Fourier transform of a band-limited function. This filter was used by Bracewell and Riddle [6, 8]) as well as by Ramachandran and Lakshminarayanan [44].

- The *Shepp–Logan filter*:

$$A_3(\omega) = |\omega| \cdot \left(\frac{\sin(\pi\omega/(2L))}{\pi\omega/(2L)} \right) \cdot \sqcap_L(\omega)$$

$$= \begin{cases} \frac{2L}{\pi} \cdot |\sin(\pi\omega/(2L))| & \text{if } |\omega| \leq L, \\ 0 & \text{if } |\omega| > L. \end{cases} \tag{7.28}$$

This filter was introduced by Shepp and Logan [49].

- The *low-pass cosine filter*:

$$A_2(\omega) = |\omega| \cdot \cos(\pi\omega/(2L)) \cdot \sqcap_L(\omega)$$

$$= \begin{cases} |\omega| \cos(\pi\omega/(2L)) & \text{if } |\omega| \leq L, \\ 0 & \text{if } |\omega| > L. \end{cases} \tag{7.29}$$

This filter is commonly used in signal analysis.

We conclude this chapter by looking at the general form of a band-limited function. So, let f be band-limited and select a number $L > 0$ such that $\mathcal{F}f(\omega) = 0$ whenever $|\omega| > L$. In particular, this means that there is some function G such that

$$\mathcal{F}f(\omega) = \sqcap_L(\omega) \cdot G(\omega),$$

where, again, $\sqcap_L(\omega) = 1$ when $|\omega| \leq L$ and $\sqcap_L(\omega) = 0$ when $|\omega| > L$. From Example 5.16 and Theorem 5.12, we know that $\sqcap_L$ is the Fourier transform of the function $\phi(x) = \sin(Lx)/(\pi x)$. If we let $g = \mathcal{F}^{-1}G$, then we see that $\mathcal{F}f = \mathcal{F}\phi \cdot \mathcal{F}g$, the product of two Fourier transforms. Hence, from Theorem 7.9, it follows that $\mathcal{F}f = \mathcal{F}(\phi * g)$ and, hence that $f = \phi * g$. This is therefore the general form that a band-limited function must have: the convolution of the function ϕ, for some value of L, with an integrable function g.

7.9   Exercises

1. Use a computer algebra system to compute and plot the convolutions of various pairs of functions. (Note: It is perfectly reasonable to form the convolution of a function with itself !)

2. In this exercise, let the filter function be $\sqcap_{1/2}$. (Recall that $\sqcap_{\frac{1}{2}}(x) = 1$ for $-1/2 \leq x \leq 1/2$ and $\sqcap_{1/2}(x) = 0$ when $|x| > 1/2$.)

    (a) For $g(x) = \cos(x)$, compute $(\sqcap_{1/2} * g)(x)$ for x real.
    (b) For $h(x) = \sin(x)$, compute $(\sqcap_{1/2} * h)(x)$ for x real.
    (c) For $F(x) = e^{-|x|}$, compute $(\sqcap_{1/2} * F)(x)$ for x real.

3. Suppose the function f vanishes outside the interval $[a, b]$ and the function g vanishes outside the interval $[c, d]$. Show that the convolution $f * g$ vanishes outside the interval $[a + c, b + d]$.

4. Apply the inverse Fourier transform $\mathcal{F}^{-1}$ to both sides of (7.13) and (7.14) to provide companion statements about the inverse Fourier transform of a convolution and of a product.

5. Apply the Rayleigh-Plancherel Theorem 7.11 to the function $f(x) = e^{-|x|}$ in order to evaluate the integral

$$\int_{-\infty}^{\infty} \frac{1}{\left(1 + \omega^2\right)^2} \, d\omega \, .$$

(*Note:* One can evaluate this integral by hand, but it's much easier to evaluate the companion integral in the Theorem!)

6. Show that, if f and g are suitable functions of two real variables, then

$$\mathcal{R}(f * g)(t, \, \theta) = (\mathcal{R}f * \mathcal{R}g)(t, \, \theta) \tag{7.30}$$

for all values of t and θ. (*Hint:* This can be proven either as a consequence of the central slice theorem (Theorem 6.1) or directly from the definitions, using (7.16) and (7.17).)

7. Set $f(x, y) = \delta(x, y) = \delta(x) \cdot \delta(y)$ in either Proposition 7.20 or Exercise 6 above. What does this suggest about the value of $\mathcal{R}\delta(t, \theta)$?

8. (a) Compute the FWHM (full width half maximum) of the Lorentzian signal

$$g(\omega) = \frac{T_2}{1 + 4\pi^2 T_2^2 (\omega - \omega_0)^2},$$

where T_2 is a constant (one of the *relaxation constants* related to magnetic resonance imaging) and the signal is centered around the angular frequency ω_0.

(b) Find a value for B so that the Gaussian signal

$$f(\omega) = T_2 e^{-B(\omega - \omega_0)^2}$$

has the same FWHM as the Lorentzian signal in part (a).

(c) For several values of the relaxation constant T_2, plot and compare the graphs of the signals in parts (a) and (b).

9. In section 7.3 above, we said the following.

[T]he smallest distance between distinct features ... in the signal S that will still be distinct in the filtered signal $(\phi * S)$ is $a = \text{FWHM}(\phi)$.

(a) Experiment with this using a signal S made up of two narrow tent functions and a filter ϕ in the shape of a box function. Try a variety of widths for the box. (As mentioned in the text, take FWHM to be the width of the box.) Convince yourself that if the box is wide enough, then it can capture both tents at once when we slide it along to form the convolution.

(b) Experiment some more with a signal S consisting of a few cycles of a cosine wave and a filter ϕ in the form of a tent. Are the crests of the original cosine wave still distinct in the convolution?

8

Discrete Image Reconstruction

8.1 Introduction

We have seen that, when complete continuous X-ray data are available, then an attenuation-coefficient function $f(x, y)$ can be reconstructed exactly using the filtered back-projection formula, Theorem 6.2. To repeat,

$$f(x, y) = \frac{1}{2}\mathcal{B}\left\{\mathcal{F}^{-1}\left[\,|S|\,\mathcal{F}\,(\mathcal{R}f)\,(S,\,\theta)\right]\right\}(x, y). \tag{8.1}$$

In Chapter 7, section 7.8, we discussed the practice of replacing the absolute-value function $|\cdot|$ in (8.1) with a low-pass filter A, obtained by multiplying the absolute value by a window function that vanishes outside some finite interval. Then, in place of (8.1), we use the approximation

$$f(x, y) \approx \frac{1}{2}\mathcal{B}\left(\mathcal{F}^{-1}A * \mathcal{R}f\right)(x, y). \tag{8.2}$$

The starting point in the implementation of (8.2) in the practical reconstruction of images from X-ray data is that only a finite number of values of $\mathcal{R}f(S, \theta)$ are available in a real study. This raises both questions of accuracy — *How many values are needed in order to generate a clinically useful image?* — and problems of computation — *What do the various components of the formula (8.2) mean in a discrete setting?* Also, as we shall see, one step in the algorithm requires essentially that we fill in some missing values. This is done using a process called interpolation that we will discuss later. Each different method of interpolation has its advantages and disadvantages. And, of course, the choice of the low-pass filter affects image quality. (See [45] and [48], from the early days of CT, for concise discussions of these issues.)

Electronic supplementary material The online version of this chapter (doi: 10.1007/978-3-319-22665-1_8) contains supplementary material, which is available to authorized users.

T.G. Feeman, *The Mathematics of Medical Imaging*, Springer Undergraduate
Texts in Mathematics and Technology, DOI 10.1007/978-3-319-22665-1_8

8.2 Sampling

The term *sampling* refers to the situation where the values of a function that presumably is defined on the whole real line are known or are computed only at a discrete set of points. For instance, we might know the values of the function at all points of the form $k \cdot \tau$, where τ is called the *sample spacing*. The basic problem is to determine how many sampled values are enough, or what value τ should have, to form an accurate description of the function as a whole.

For example, consider a string of sampled values $\{f(k) = 1\}$, sampled at every integer (so $\tau = 1$). These could be the values of the constant function $f(x) \equiv 1$, or of the periodic function $\cos(2\pi x)$. If it is the latter, then we obviously would need more samples to be certain.

Heuristically, we might think of a signal as consisting of a compilation of sine or cosine waves of various frequencies and amplitudes. The narrowest bump in this compilation constitutes the smallest feature that is present in the signal and corresponds to the wave that has the shortest wavelength. The reciprocal of the shortest wavelength present in the signal is the maximum frequency that is present in the Fourier transform of the signal. So this signal is a *band-limited* function — its Fourier transform is zero outside a finite interval.

Now, suppose that f is a band-limited function for which $\mathcal{F}f(\omega) = 0$ whenever $|\omega| > L$. By definition (see (4.7)), the *Fourier series coefficients* of $\mathcal{F}f$ are given by

$$C_n = \left(\frac{1}{2L}\right) \int_{-L}^{L} \mathcal{F}f(\omega)\, e^{-i\pi n\omega/L}\, d\omega \,, \tag{8.3}$$

where n is any integer. (Here, we are acting as if $\mathcal{F}f$ has been extended beyond the interval $[-L, L]$ to be periodic on the real line, with period $2L$.) For each integer n, then,

$$(2\pi) \cdot f(\pi n/L) = 2\pi \cdot \mathcal{F}^{-1}(\mathcal{F}f)(\pi n/L)$$

$$= \int_{-\infty}^{\infty} \mathcal{F}f(\omega)\, e^{i\omega\pi n/L}\, d\omega$$

$$= \int_{-L}^{L} \mathcal{F}f(\omega)\, e^{i\omega\pi n/L}\, d\omega \ \ \text{since } f \text{ is band-limited}$$

$$= (2L) \cdot C_{-n}.$$

That is,

$$C_{-n} = (\pi/L) \cdot f(\pi n/L) \text{ for every integer } n.$$

Assuming that $\mathcal{F}f$ is continuous, it follows from standard results of Fourier series that

$$\mathcal{F}f(\omega) = \sum_{n=-\infty}^{\infty} C_{-n}\, e^{-in\pi\omega/L} = \left(\frac{\pi}{L}\right) \cdot \sum_{n=-\infty}^{\infty} f(\pi n/L)\, e^{-in\pi\omega/L}. \tag{8.4}$$

Finally, all of this means that, for every x, we have

$$f(x) = \mathcal{F}^{-1}(\mathcal{F}f)(x)$$

$$= \left(\frac{1}{2\pi}\right) \int_{-L}^{L} \mathcal{F}f(\omega)\, e^{i\omega x}\, dx$$

$$= \left(\frac{1}{2\pi}\right)\left(\frac{\pi}{L}\right) \int_{-L}^{L} \left[\sum_{n=-\infty}^{\infty} f(\pi n/L)\, e^{-in\pi\omega/L}\right] e^{i\omega x}\, dx \text{ from (8.4)}$$

$$= \left(\frac{1}{2L}\right) \sum_{n=-\infty}^{\infty} \left[f(\pi n/L) \cdot \int_{-L}^{L} e^{i\omega(Lx-n\pi)/L}\, d\omega\right]$$

$$= \left(\frac{1}{2L}\right) \sum_{n=-\infty}^{\infty} f(\pi n/L) \cdot (2L) \cdot \left(\frac{\sin(Lx - n\pi)}{Lx - n\pi}\right) \text{ (Ch. 4, Exer. 4)}$$

$$= \sum_{n=-\infty}^{\infty} f(\pi n/L) \cdot \left(\frac{\sin(Lx - n\pi)}{Lx - n\pi}\right).$$

Thus we see that, for a band-limited function f whose Fourier transform vanishes outside the interval $[-L, L]$, the function f can be reconstructed exactly from the values $\{f(n\pi/L) : -\infty < n < \infty\}$. In other words, the appropriate sample spacing for the function f is $\tau = \pi/L$. Since L represents the maximum value of $|\omega|$ present in the Fourier transform $\mathcal{F}f$, the value $2\pi/L$ represents the smallest wavelength present in the signal f. Therefore, *the optimal sample spacing is equal to half of the size of the smallest detail present in the signal.* This result is known as *Nyquist's theorem* and the value $\tau = \pi/L$ is called the *Nyquist distance*.

To sum up, we have established the following.

Theorem 8.1. Nyquist's theorem. *If f is a square-integrable band-limited function such that the Fourier transform $\mathcal{F}f(\omega) = 0$ whenever $|\omega| > L$, then, for every real number x,*

$$f(x) = \sum_{n=-\infty}^{\infty} f(\pi n/L) \cdot \frac{\sin(Lx - n\pi)}{Lx - n\pi}. \tag{8.5}$$

Nyquist's theorem is also sometimes referred to as *Shannon–Whittaker interpolation* since it asserts that *any* value of the function f can be interpolated from the values $\{f(n\pi/L)\}$.

A heuristic approach to Nyquist's theorem. As above, assume that the function f is band-limited, with $\mathcal{F}f(\omega) = 0$ whenever $|\omega| > L$. We want to extend $\mathcal{F}f$ to be periodic on the whole line, so we can take the period to be $2L$, the length of the interval $-L \leq \omega \leq L$. Now, each of the functions $\omega \mapsto e^{-in\pi\omega/L}$, where n is an integer, has period $2L$. From the definition of the Fourier transform,

$$\mathcal{F}f(\omega) = \int_{x=-\infty}^{\infty} f(x)\, e^{-i\omega x}\, dx. \tag{8.6}$$

Approximate this integral using a Riemann sum with $dx = \pi/L$. That is, the Riemann sum will use a partition of the line that includes all points of the form $n\pi/L$, where n is an integer. This results in the approximation

$$\mathcal{F}f(\omega) \approx \left(\frac{\pi}{L}\right) \cdot \sum_{n=-\infty}^{\infty} f(n\pi/L)\, e^{-in\pi\omega/L}.$$

This approximates $\mathcal{F}f$ in a way that is periodic on the whole line with period $2L$. Notice that this is the same as (8.4) except for having "$\approx$" instead of "$=$." In the proof above, we appealed to results in the theory of Fourier series that assert that this approximation is actually an equality. Without that knowledge, we instead substitute the approximation for $\mathcal{F}f$ into the rest of the proof of Nyquist's theorem and end up with the approximation

$$f(x) \approx \sum_{n=-\infty}^{\infty} f(\pi n/L) \cdot \frac{\sin(Lx - n\pi)}{Lx - n\pi}. \tag{8.7}$$

Nyquist's theorem, which builds on the results concerning Fourier series, asserts that this is in fact an equality.

Oversampling. The interpolation formula (8.5) is an infinite series. In practice, we would only use a partial sum. However, the series (8.5) may converge fairly slowly because the expression $\sin(Lx - n\pi)/(Lx - n\pi)$ is on the order of $(1/n)$ for large values of n and the harmonic series $\sum 1/n$ diverges. That means that a partial sum might require a large number of terms in order to achieve a good approximation to $f(x)$.

To address this difficulty, notice that, if $\mathcal{F}f(\omega) = 0$ whenever $|\omega| > L$, and if $R > L$, then $\mathcal{F}f(\omega) = 0$ whenever $|\omega| > R$ as well. Thus, we can use Shannon–Whittaker interpolation on the interval $[-R, R]$ instead of $[-L, L]$. This requires that we sample the function f at the Nyquist distance π/R, instead of π/L. Since $\pi/R < \pi/L$, this results in what is called *oversampling* of the function f. So there is a computational price to pay for oversampling, but the improvement in the results, when using a partial sum to approximate $f(x)$, may be worth that price.

8.3 Discrete low-pass filters

The image reconstruction formula (8.2) involves the inverse Fourier transform $\mathcal{F}^{-1}A$ for the low-pass filter A. In practice, this, too, will be sampled, just like the Radon transform. Nyquist's theorem, Theorem 8.1, tells us how many sampled values are needed to get an accurate representation of $\mathcal{F}^{-1}A$. Here, we investigate how this works for two particular low-pass filters.

Example 8.2. The *Shepp–Logan filter*, introduced in (7.28), is defined by

$$A(\omega) = |\omega| \cdot \left(\frac{\sin(\pi\omega/(2L))}{\pi\omega/(2L)} \right) \cdot \sqcap_L(\omega)$$

$$= \begin{cases} \frac{2L}{\pi} \cdot |\sin(\pi\omega/(2L))| & \text{if } |\omega| \leq L, \\ 0 & \text{if } |\omega| > L, \end{cases} \tag{8.8}$$

for some choice of $L > 0$.

Since A vanishes outside the interval $[-L, L]$, the inverse Fourier transform of A is a band-limited function. From the fact that A is also an even function, we compute, for each real number x,

$$(\mathcal{F}^{-1}A)(x) = \frac{1}{\pi} \int_0^L \frac{2L}{\pi} \cdot \sin(\pi\omega/(2L)) \cdot \cos(x\omega) \, d\omega$$

$$= \left(\frac{L}{\pi^2} \right) \cdot \left\{ \frac{\cos((x - \pi/(2L))\omega)}{x - \pi/(2L)} - \frac{\cos((x + \pi/(2L))\omega)}{x + \pi/(2L)} \right\} \Bigg|_0^L$$

$$= \left(\frac{L}{\pi^2} \right) \cdot \left\{ \left[\frac{\cos(Lx - \pi/2)}{x - \pi/(2L)} - \frac{\cos(Lx + \pi/2)}{x + \pi/(2L)} \right] \right.$$

$$\left. - \left[\frac{1}{x - \pi/(2L)} - \frac{1}{x + \pi/(2L)} \right] \right\} . \tag{8.9}$$

According to Nyquist's theorem, the function $\mathcal{F}^{-1}A$ can be reconstructed exactly from its values taken in increments of the Nyquist distance π/L. Setting $x = \pi n/L$ in (8.9) yields

$$(\mathcal{F}^{-1}A)(\pi n/L) = \left(\frac{L}{\pi^2} \right) \cdot \left\{ \left[\frac{\cos(\pi n - \pi/2)}{\pi n/L - \pi/(2L)} - \frac{\cos(\pi n + \pi/2)}{\pi n/L + \pi/(2L)} \right] \right.$$

$$\left. - \left[\frac{1}{\pi n/L - \pi/(2L)} - \frac{1}{\pi n/L + \pi/(2L)} \right] \right\}$$

$$= \left(\frac{L}{\pi^2} \right) \cdot \left\{ \frac{1}{\pi n/L + \pi/(2L)} - \frac{1}{\pi n/L - \pi/(2L)} \right\}$$

$$= \frac{4L^2}{\pi^3 (1 - 4n^2)} . \tag{8.10}$$

Example 8.3. The *Ram–Lak filter*, defined in (7.27), has the formula

$$A(\omega) = |\omega| \cdot \sqcap_L(\omega) = \begin{cases} |\omega| & \text{if } |\omega| \leq L, \\ 0 & \text{if } |\omega| > L. \end{cases} \tag{8.11}$$

Proceeding as in the previous example, we find that the inverse Fourier transform of the Ram–Lak filter satisfies

$$(\mathcal{F}^{-1}A)(x) = \frac{1}{\pi} \int_0^L \omega \cdot \cos(x\omega)\, d\omega$$

$$= \left(\frac{1}{\pi}\right) \cdot \left\{ \frac{\cos(x\omega) + (x\omega) \cdot \sin(x\omega)}{x^2} \right\} \Bigg|_0^L$$

$$= \left(\frac{1}{\pi}\right) \cdot \left\{ \frac{\cos(Lx) + (Lx) \cdot \sin(Lx) - 1}{x^2} \right\}$$

$$= \left(\frac{1}{\pi}\right) \cdot \left\{ \frac{(Lx) \cdot \sin(Lx)}{x^2} - \frac{2 \cdot \sin^2(Lx/2)}{x^2} \right\}, \tag{8.12}$$

where the trigonometric identity $\cos(\theta) = 1 - 2 \cdot \sin^2(\theta/2)$ was used in the last step.

As before, set $x = \pi n/L$ to evaluate $\mathcal{F}^{-1}A$ at multiples of the Nyquist distance π/L. Thus,

$$(\mathcal{F}^{-1}A)(\pi n/L) = \left(\frac{1}{\pi}\right) \cdot \left\{ \frac{(\pi n) \cdot \sin(\pi n)}{(\pi n/L)^2} - \frac{2 \cdot \sin^2(\pi n/2)}{(\pi n/L)^2} \right\}$$

$$= \frac{L^2}{2\pi} \cdot \left\{ \frac{2 \cdot \sin(\pi n)}{\pi n} - \left[\frac{\sin(\pi n/2)}{(\pi n/2)} \right]^2 \right\}. \tag{8.13}$$

For $n = 0$, the right-hand side of (8.13) makes sense only as a limit. This gives the value $(\mathcal{F}^{-1}A)(0) = L^2/(2\pi)$. For nonzero even integers n, (8.13) simplifies to $(\mathcal{F}^{-1}A)(\pi n/L) = 0$. When n is odd, the value is given by $(\mathcal{F}^{-1}A)(\pi n/L) = -2L^2/(\pi^3 \cdot n^2)$. Figure 8.1 provides a comparison of the discrete inverse Fourier transforms of the Ram–Lak and Shepp–Logan low-pass filters, using $L = 10$ and sampling the inverse Fourier transforms at the Nyquist distance $\pi/10$.

Example 8.4. The low-pass cosine filter, defined in (7.29), is left for the exercises.

Example with R 8.5. In the preceding examples, we computed the discrete inverse Fourier Transforms for the Shepp–Logan and Ram–Lak low-pass filters. It is easy enough to record this in R. Then we evaluate at a set of points and draw the plot, like so.

```
L=10.0 #sets the window
xval=(pi/L)*(-L:L) #sample at Nyquist dist.
##Inverse Fourier transform of the Ram-Lak filter:
IFRL=-function(n){
ifelse(n==0,(0.5)*L^2/pi,
((0.5)*L^2/pi)*(2*sin(pi*n)/(pi*n)-(sin(pi*n/2)/(pi*n/2))
   ^2))}
yval1=IFRL(-L:L)
##Inverse Fourier transform of the Shepp-Logan (sinc)
   filter:
IFSL=function(n){
(4*L^2/pi^3)*(1/(1-4*n^2))}
```

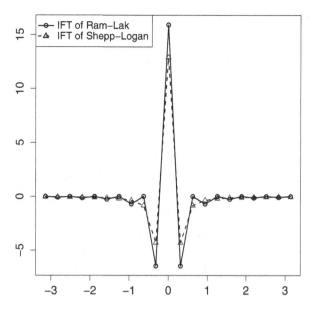

Fig. 8.1. Comparison of the discrete inverse Fourier transforms of the Shepp–Logan and Ram–Lak low-pass filters, from values sampled at the Nyquist distance π/L, with $L = 10$.

```
yval2=IFSL(-L:L)
### plot ##
plot(xval,yval1,pch=1,lwd=2,xlab="",ylab="")
lines(xval,yval1,lwd=2,lty=1,add=T)
points(xval,yval2,pch=2)
lines(xval,yval2,lwd=2,lty=2)
```

8.4   Discrete Radon transform

In the context of a CT scan, the X-ray machine does not assess the attenuation along every line $\ell_{t,\theta}$. Instead, in the model we have been using, the Radon transform is sampled for a finite number of angles θ between 0 and π and, at each of these angles, for some finite number of values of t. Both the angles and the t values are evenly spaced. So, in this model, the X-ray sources rotate by a fixed angle from one set of readings to the next and, within each setting, the individual X-ray beams are evenly spaced. This is called the *parallel beam geometry*.

If the machine takes scans at N different angles, incremented by $d\theta = \pi/N$, then the specific values of θ that occur are $\{k\pi/N : 0 \leq k \leq N - 1\}$. We are assuming that the beams at each angle form a set of parallel lines. The spacing between these beams, say τ, is called the *sample spacing*. For instance, suppose there are $2 \cdot M + 1$ parallel X-ray beams at each angle. With the object to be scanned centered at the origin, the corresponding values of t are $\{j \cdot \tau \, : \, -M \leq j \leq M\}$. (The specific values of M and τ essentially depend on the design of the machine itself and on the sizes of the objects the machine is designed to scan.) Thus, the continuous Radon transform $\mathcal{R}f$ is replaced by the discrete function $\mathcal{R}_D f$ defined, for $-M \leq j \leq M$ and $0 \leq k \leq (N-1)$, by

$$\mathcal{R}_D f_{j,k} = \mathcal{R}f(j\tau, k\pi/N). \tag{8.14}$$

Example with R 8.6. In Examples 2.13 and 2.15, in Chapter 2, we used R to compute and display sinograms for a variety of phantoms. Since R is a discrete programming environment by design, we were actually computing the discrete Radon transform of each phantom. Indeed, our first step was to define the sets of values for both t and θ to be included in the scan. Then we created a vector whose entries were the values $\mathcal{R}_D f_{j,k}$ for all j and k.

To implement formula (8.2), we must now decide what we mean by the convolution of two functions for which we have only sampled values. At the same time, we will adopt some rules and conventions for dealing with discretely defined functions in general.

8.5 Discrete functions and convolution

A discrete function of one variable is a mapping from the integers into the set of real or complex numbers. In other words, a discrete function g may be thought of as a two-way infinite list, or sequence, of real or complex numbers $\{\ldots, g(-2), g(-1), g(0), g(1), g(2), \ldots\}$. Because of this connection to sequences, we will often write g_n instead of $g(n)$ to designate the value of a discrete function g at the integer n.

Remark 8.7. Most of the discrete functions considered here arise by taking a continuous function, say g, and evaluating it at a discrete set of values, say $\{x_n \, : \, n \in \mathbb{Z}\}$. The subscript notation allows us to denote the discrete function also by g, with $g_n = g(x_n)$. The definition of the discrete Radon transform, in (8.14), is an example of this notation.

Definition 8.8. In analogy with the integral that defines continuous convolution, the *discrete convolution* of two discrete functions f and g, denoted by $f \bar{*} g$, is defined by

$$(f \bar{*} g)_m = \sum_{j=-\infty}^{\infty} f_j \cdot g_{(m-j)} \quad \text{for each integer } m. \tag{8.15}$$

As with infinite integrals, there is the issue, which we evade for the time being, of whether this sum converges.

Proposition 8.9. *A few properties of discrete convolution are*

(i) $f \bar{*} g = g \bar{*} f$,

(ii) $f \bar{*} (g + h) = f \bar{*} g + f \bar{*} h$, *and*

(iii) $f \bar{*} (\alpha g) = \alpha (f \bar{*} g)$,

for suitable functions f, g, *and* h, *and for any constant* α.

In practice, we typically know the values of a function f only at a finite set of points, say $\{k \cdot \tau : k = 0, 1, \ldots, (N-1)\}$, where N is the total number of points at which f has been computed and τ is the sample spacing. For simplicity, let $f_k = f(k\tau)$ for each k between 0 and $(N-1)$ and use the set of values $\{f_1, f_2, \ldots, f_{N-1}\}$ to represent f as a discrete function. There are two useful ways to extend this sequence to one that is defined for all integers. The simplest approach is just to pad the sequence with zeros by setting $f_k = 0$ whenever k is not between 0 and $N-1$. Another intriguing and useful idea is to extend the sequence to be *periodic* with period N. Specifically, for any given integer m, there is a unique integer n such that $0 \leq m + n \cdot N \leq (N-1)$. We *define* $f_m = f_{m+n\cdot N}$. Thus, $f_N = f_0, f_{-1} = f_{N-1}, f_{N+1} = f_1$, and so on. This defines the discrete function $f = \{f_k\}$ as a periodic function on the set of all integers. We will refer to such a function as an N-*periodic discrete function*.

Definition 8.10. For two N-periodic discrete functions $f = \{f_k : 0 \leq k \leq N-1\}$ and $g = \{g_k : 0 \leq k \leq N-1\}$, the *discrete convolution*, denoted as before by $f \bar{*} g$, is defined by

$$(f \bar{*} g)_m := \sum_{j=0}^{N-1} f_j \cdot g_{(m-j)} \text{ for each integer } m. \tag{8.16}$$

This is obviously similar to Definition 8.8 except that the sum extends only over one full period rather than the full set of integers. Notice that when m and j satisfy $0 \leq m, j \leq (N-1)$, then the difference $(m-j)$ satisfies $|m-j| \leq (N-1)$. The periodicity of the discrete functions enables us to assign values to the discrete convolution function at points outside the range 0 to $(N-1)$, so that $f \bar{*} g$ also has period N.

The two versions of discrete convolution in (8.15) and (8.16) can be reconciled if one of the two functions has only finitely many nonzero values.

Proposition 8.11. *Let* f *and* g *be two-way infinite discrete functions and suppose there is some natural number* K *such that* $g_k = 0$ *whenever* $k < 0$ *or* $k \geq K$. *Let* M *be an integer satisfying* $M \geq K - 1$ *and let* $\widetilde{f}$ *and* $\widetilde{g}$ *be the* $(2M+1)$-*periodic discrete functions defined by* $\widetilde{f}(m) = f(m)$ *and* $\widetilde{g}(m) = g(m)$ *for* $-M \leq m \leq M$. *Then, for all* m *satisfying* $0 \leq m \leq K - 1$,

$$(f \bar{*} g)_m = \left(\widetilde{f} \bar{*} \widetilde{g}\right)(m). \tag{8.17}$$

Proof. Let f, g, K, M, $\widetilde{f}$, and $\widetilde{g}$ be as stated. For each pair of integers m and j satisfying $0 \leq m, j \leq K - 1$, it follows that $|m - j| \leq K - 1$. Thus, since $M \geq K - 1$, we get that $f(m - j) = \widetilde{f}(m - j)$. Now fix a value of m with $0 \leq m \leq K - 1$. From the definition (8.15) and the properties of $\bar{*}$, we have

$$(f \bar{*} g)_m = \sum_{j=-\infty}^{\infty} f(m - j) \cdot g(j)$$

$$= \sum_{j=0}^{K-1} f(m-j) \cdot g(j)$$

$$= \sum_{j=0}^{K-1} \widetilde{f}(m-j) \cdot g(j)$$

$$= \sum_{j=-M}^{M} \widetilde{f}(m-j) \cdot \widetilde{g}(j)$$

$$= \left(\widetilde{f} \,\widetilde{*}\, \widetilde{g}\right)(m).$$

□

What is really going on in this proposition? Well, there are a few worries when it comes to using periodic discrete functions. One concern is that it may not be clear what the appropriate period is. So, we might sample a finite set of values of a continuous periodic function, but the values we compute might not correspond to a full period. Then, when we extend the data to form a discrete periodic function, we have the wrong one. Or, the function whose values we have sampled might not be periodic at all. Then we ought not to use a periodic discrete function to model it. The proposition offers a remedy that is known as *zero padding*: we can take a finite set of values of a function (g) and, by padding the sequence of values with a lot of zeros, form a periodic discrete function ($\widetilde{g}$) in such a way that the periodic discrete convolution gives the same value as the true discrete convolution, at least at the points where the value has been sampled.

For an illustration of the benefits of zero padding, consider the function $\sqcap_{1/2}$ defined, as before, by

$$\sqcap_{1/2}(x) = \begin{cases} 1 & \text{if } -1/2 \le x < 1/2, \\ 0 & \text{otherwise.} \end{cases}$$

Suppose we sample $\sqcap_{1/2}$ at two points $x = -1/2$ and $x = 0$ and, so generate the 2-periodic discrete function f with $f_0 = f_1 = 1$. For the periodic discrete convolution $f \widetilde{*} f$, we get

$$(f \widetilde{*} f)_0 = 1 \cdot 1 + 1 \cdot 1 = 2 \text{ and}$$

$$(f \widetilde{*} f)_1 = 1 \cdot 1 + 1 \cdot 1 = 2.$$

Now pad the function f with a couple of zeros to get the 4-periodic function $\widetilde{f} = \{1, 1, 0, 0\}$. (We could also think of this as sampling the function $\sqcap_{1/2}$ at the x values $-1/2, 0, 1/2$, and 1.) Then we get

$$(\widetilde{f} \widetilde{*} \widetilde{f})_0 = 1 \cdot 1 + 1 \cdot 0 + 0 \cdot 0 + 0 \cdot 1 = 1,$$

$$(\widetilde{f} \widetilde{*} \widetilde{f})_1 = 1 \cdot 1 + 1 \cdot 1 + 0 \cdot 0 + 0 \cdot 0 = 2,$$

$$\left(\widetilde{f} \mathbin{\widetilde{*}} \widetilde{f}\right)_2 = 1 \cdot 0 + 1 \cdot 1 + 0 \cdot 1 + 0 \cdot 1 = 1 \ , \text{ and}$$

$$\left(\widetilde{f} \mathbin{\widetilde{*}} \widetilde{f}\right)_3 = 1 \cdot 0 + 1 \cdot 0 + 0 \cdot 1 + 0 \cdot 1 = 0.$$

Instead of accurately representing $\sqcap_{1/2}$, the function f acts like a constant, and so $f \mathbin{\widetilde{*}} f$ is constant, too. But $\widetilde{f}$ does a better job of representing $\sqcap_{1/2}$, and the convolution $\widetilde{f} \mathbin{\widetilde{*}} \widetilde{f}$ is a discrete version of the function $2(\sqcap_{1/2} * \sqcap_{1/2}) = 2(1 - |x|)$, for $-1 \le x < 1$, sampled at the x values $-1/2, 0, 1/2$, and 1.

Importantly, Proposition 8.11 applies to the discrete convolution of a sampled version of the band-limited function $\mathcal{F}^{-1}A$, where A is a low-pass filter, and the discrete (sampled) Radon transform $\mathcal{R}_D f$, where f is the attenuation function we wish to reconstruct. Since the scanned object is finite in size, we can set $\mathcal{R}_D f(j, \theta) = 0$ whenever $|j|$ is sufficiently large. Thus, with enough zero padding, the discrete Radon transform (8.14) can be extended to be periodic in the radial variable ($j\tau$), and (8.17) shows how to compute the desired discrete convolution.

For discrete functions defined using polar coordinates, the discrete convolution is carried out in the radial variable only. In particular, for a given filter A, we compute the discrete convolution of the sampled inverse Fourier transform of A with the discrete Radon transform of f as

$$\left(\mathcal{F}^{-1}A \mathbin{\widetilde{*}} \mathcal{R}_D f\right)_{m, \theta} = \sum_{j=0}^{N-1} \left(\mathcal{F}^{-1}A\right)_j \cdot \left(\mathcal{R}_D f\right)_{m-j, \theta} . \tag{8.18}$$

Example with R 8.12. In Example 7.15, in Chapter 7, we applied the `convolve` procedure in R to compute the back projection of the Radon transform of a function. As mentioned there, this procedure is inherently a discrete convolution, provided one remembers to flip one of the two discrete functions involved. The option `type` `="open"` that we used in that example applies zero padding to the sequences before computing the convolution. In the next section, we will apply `convolve` as one step in the implementation of the filtered back projection formula (8.2).

8.6   Discrete Fourier transform

For a continuous function f, the Fourier transform is defined by

$$\mathcal{F}f(\omega) = \int_{-\infty}^{\infty} f(x)\, e^{-i\omega x}\, dx$$

for every real number ω. For a discrete analogue to this, we consider an N-periodic discrete function f. Replacing the integral in the Fourier transform by a sum and summing over one full period of f yields the expression

$$\sum_{k=0}^{N-1} f_k\, e^{-i\omega k}.$$

Now take ω to have the form $\omega_j = 2\pi j/N$. Then, for each choice of k, we get $e^{-i\omega_j k} = e^{-i2\pi kj/N}$. This is a periodic function with period N in the j variable, just as f_k has period N in the k variable. In this way, the Fourier transform of the discrete function f is also a discrete function, defined for ω_j, with $j = 0, 1, \ldots, (N-1)$, and extended by periodicity to every integer.

Definition 8.13. The *discrete Fourier transform*, denoted by $\mathcal{F}_D$, transforms an N-periodic discrete function f into another N-periodic discrete function $\mathcal{F}_D f$ defined by

$$(\mathcal{F}_D f)_j = \sum_{k=0}^{N-1} f_k\, e^{-i2\pi kj/N} \quad \text{for } j = 0, 1, \ldots, (N-1). \tag{8.19}$$

For other integer values of j, the value of $(\mathcal{F}_D f)_j$ is defined by the periodicity requirement.

Remark 8.14. In the summation (8.19), we can replace the range $0 \le k \le (N-1)$ by any string of the form $M \le k \le (M+N-1)$, where M is an integer. This is due to the periodicity of the discrete function f.

Example 8.15. Fix a natural number M and set

$$f_k = \begin{cases} 1 & \text{if } -M \le k \le M, \\ 0 & \text{otherwise.} \end{cases}$$

Now let $N > 2M$ and think of f as being an N-periodic discrete function. (Thus, f consists of a string of 1s possibly padded with some 0 s.) We might think of f as a discrete sampling of the characteristic function of a finite interval. The continuous Fourier transform of a characteristic function is a function of the form $a\sin(bx)/x$.

In the discrete setting, use the periodicity of f to compute, for each $j = 0, 1, \ldots, N-1$,

$$(\mathcal{F}_D f)_j = \sum_{k=0}^{M} e^{-2\pi i kj/N} + \sum_{k=N-M}^{N-1} e^{-2\pi i kj/N}$$

$$= e^0 + \sum_{k=1}^{M} \left(e^{-2\pi i kj/N} + e^{-2\pi i (N-k)j/N} \right)$$

$$= 1 + 2 \cdot \sum_{k=1}^{M} \cos(2\pi kj/N)$$

$$= 2 \cdot (1/2 + \cos(2\pi j/N) + \cos(2\pi 2j/N) + \cdots + \cos(2\pi Mj/N))$$

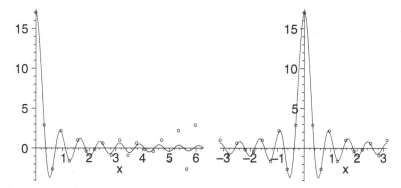

Fig. 8.2. Continuous and discrete Fourier transforms of a square wave. Zero padding has been used in the sampling of the square wave. The wrap around in the second picture illustrates the N-periodic behavior of the discrete transform.

$$= 2 \cdot \frac{\sin\left((M + 1/2) \cdot 2\pi j/N\right)}{2 \cdot \sin(\pi j/N)}$$

$$= \frac{\sin\left((2M + 1)\pi j/N\right)}{\sin(\pi j/N)}.$$

We have used the identity

$$1/2 + \cos(\theta) + \cos(2\theta) + \cdots + \cos(M\theta) = \frac{\sin((M + 1/2)\theta)}{2 \cdot \sin(\theta/2)}. \tag{8.20}$$

Figure 8.2 shows a comparison, with $M = 8$ and $N = 20$, of the graph of

$$y = \frac{\sin((2 \cdot M + 1)x/2)}{x/2}$$

with the set of points

$$\left(2\pi j/N, \frac{\sin\left((2 \cdot M + 1)\pi j/N\right)}{\sin(\pi j/N)}\right),$$

where the point $(0, (2 \cdot M + 1))$ corresponds to $j = 0$. The diagram on the left shows the situation for $0 \le x \le 2\pi$ and $j = 0, 1, \ldots, N - 1$. While the curve continues its decay, the points representing the discrete Fourier transform reveal the N-periodic behavior. In the diagram on the right, the interval is $-\pi \le x \le \pi$, corresponding to $j = -N/2, \ldots, N/2$. In comparing the two diagrams, we can see how the N-periodic behavior of the discrete Fourier transform works.

Where there is a discrete Fourier transform, there must also be an inverse transform. Indeed, the formula (8.2) demands it. To this end, we have the following.

Definition 8.16. For an N-periodic discrete function g, the *discrete inverse Fourier transform* of g is the N-periodic function defined by

$$(\mathcal{F}_D^{-1}g)_n = \frac{1}{N} \sum_{k=0}^{N-1} g_k \, e^{i2\pi kn/N}, \text{ for } n = 0, \ldots, N-1. \tag{8.21}$$

Remark 8.17. In Examples 8.2 and 8.3, in section 8.3 of this chapter, we used Nyquist's theorem, or Shannon–Whittaker interpolation, to compute samples of the inverse Fourier transforms of the Shepp–Logan and Ram–Lak low-pass filters, respectively. The filters were defined to vanish outside the interval $[-L, L]$, and, accordingly, the Nyquist distance was π/L. A funny thing happened, though, when we defined the *discrete* inverse Fourier transform, in Definition 8.16: a factor of 2π sneaked its way into the complex exponential term in the sum. To accommodate this change, the sample spacing of the N-periodic discrete function being transformed must be modified from π/L to $\pi/(2\pi L)$, or simply $1/(2L)$. What has happened is that the period of the discrete function is effectively given by setting $N = 2L$ in (8.21). Then, adding 1 to the value of n in the complex exponential changes the value of n/N by the sample spacing value $1/(2L)$; this in turn changes the value of $2\pi n/N$ by the Nyquist distance, π/L. Thus, the implied sample spacing in (8.21) is $1/N = 1/(2L)$. In other words, when we switch from the continuous version of the low-pass filter to its periodic discrete counterpart, the sampled values of the continuous inverse Fourier transform, computed at increments of the Nyquist distance π/L, correspond to sampled values of the *discrete* inverse Fourier transform computed at increments of the modified sample spacing $1/(2L)$. We will use this sample spacing in section 8.9, when we discuss the implementation of formula (8.2).

Example with R 8.18. In Example 8.5, we computed the discrete inverse Fourier Transforms for the Shepp–Logan and Ram–Lak low-pass filters. The only modification we must make to implement (8.2) is to change the size of the window to $L = 1/(2\tau)$, as just discussed, where τ is the spacing between parallel X-ray beams in the scan. Also, since the value of L is linked to the t variable, we will form a separate discrete convolution for each value of θ. We will look at this in detail in section 8.9.

The discrete analogue of the Fourier inversion theorem (Theorem 5.12) holds.

Theorem 8.19. *For a discrete function f with period N,*

$$\mathcal{F}_D^{-1}\left(\mathcal{F}_D f\right)_n = f_n \text{ for all integers } n. \tag{8.22}$$

Before we prove this theorem, we need the following fact about roots of unity.

Lemma 8.20. *For any nonzero integers M and N,*

$$\sum_{k=0}^{N-1} e^{i2\pi Mk/N} = \begin{cases} N & \textit{if } M/N \textit{ is an integer,} \\ 0 & \textit{if } M/N \textit{ is not an integer.} \end{cases} \tag{8.23}$$

Proof. If M/N is an integer, then $e^{i2\pi Mk/N} = 1$ for every integer k, whence, $\sum_{k=0}^{N-1} e^{i2\pi Mk/N} = N$.

If M/N is not an integer, then $\left(e^{i2\pi M/N}\right)^N - 1 = 0$, but $e^{i2\pi M/N} \neq 1$. Since the expression $x^N - 1$ factors as $x^N - 1 = (x-1)(1 + x + x^2 + \cdots + x^{N-1})$, it follows that

$$1 + e^{i2\pi M/N} + \left(e^{i2\pi M/N}\right)^2 + \cdots + \left(e^{i2\pi M/N}\right)^{N-1} = 0.$$

That is,

$$\sum_{k=0}^{N-1} e^{i2\pi Mk/N} = 0$$

as claimed.   □

Proof of Theorem 8.19. For a given integer n with $0 \leq n \leq (N-1)$, compute

$$\mathcal{F}_D^{-1}\left(\mathcal{F}_D f\right)_n = \frac{1}{N} \sum_{k=0}^{N-1} (\mathcal{F}_D f)_k \, e^{i2\pi kn/N}$$

$$= \frac{1}{N} \sum_{k=0}^{N-1} \left(\sum_{m=0}^{N-1} f_m \, e^{-i2\pi mk/N}\right) e^{i2\pi kn/N}$$

$$= \frac{1}{N} \sum_{m=0}^{N-1} \left[f_m \left(\sum_{k=0}^{N-1} e^{i2\pi(n-m)k/N}\right)\right].$$

When $m = n$, we have $e^{i2\pi(n-m)k/N} = 1$ for every k. So

$$\sum_{k=0}^{N-1} e^{i2\pi(n-m)k/N} = N \text{ when } m = n.$$

However, when $m \neq n$, then Lemma 8.20 asserts that

$$\sum_{k=0}^{N-1} e^{i2\pi(n-m)k/N} = 0.$$

It follows that

$$\frac{1}{N} \sum_{m=0}^{N-1} \left[f_m \left(\sum_{k=0}^{N-1} e^{i2\pi(n-m)k/N}\right)\right] = \frac{1}{N} [f_n \cdot N] = f_n .$$

That is, $\mathcal{F}_D^{-1}(\mathcal{F}_Df)_n = f_n$ for $0 \leq n \leq (N-1)$ and, by periodicity, for all integers n. □

Were we so inclined, we could establish properties about linearity, shifting, and so on for the discrete Fourier transform and its inverse. However, our focus is on the implementation of the formula (8.2) so our priority must be to study the interaction between the discrete Fourier transform and discrete convolution. In particular, the following theorem holds.

Theorem 8.21. *For two discrete functions* $f = \{f_k : 0 \leq k \leq N-1\}$ *and* $g = \{g_k : 0 \leq k \leq N-1\}$ *with the same period, we have*

$$\mathcal{F}_D(f \bar{*} g) = (\mathcal{F}_Df) \cdot (\mathcal{F}_Dg). \tag{8.24}$$

In words, the discrete Fourier transform of a convolution is the product of the discrete transforms individually.

Proof. For each integer n such that $0 \leq n \leq (N-1)$,

$$(\mathcal{F}_Df)_n \cdot (\mathcal{F}_Dg)_n$$

$$= \left(\sum_{k=0}^{N-1} f_k e^{-2\pi ink/N}\right) \cdot \left(\sum_{\ell=0}^{N-1} g_\ell e^{-2\pi in\ell/N}\right)$$

$$= \sum_{k=0}^{N-1} f_k \left(\sum_{\ell=-k}^{-k+N-1} g_\ell e^{-2\pi in\ell/N}\right) e^{-2\pi ink/N} \quad \text{(by periodicity of } g\text{)}$$

$$= \sum_{k=0}^{N-1} f_k \left(\sum_{j=0}^{N-1} g_{j-k} e^{-2\pi in(j-k)/N}\right) e^{-2\pi ink/N} \quad \text{(where } j = k + \ell\text{)}$$

$$= \sum_{j=0}^{N-1} \sum_{k=0}^{N-1} \left(f_k \cdot g_{j-k} e^{-2\pi inj/N}\right)$$

$$= \sum_{j=0}^{N-1} \left(\sum_{k=0}^{N-1} f_k \cdot g_{j-k}\right) e^{-2\pi inj/N}$$

$$= \sum_{j=0}^{N-1} (f \bar{*} g)_j e^{-2\pi inj/N}$$

$$= [\mathcal{F}_D(f \bar{*} g)]_n,$$

which is the desired result.   □

We conclude this section by mentioning a few results that are discrete versions of some of the results from earlier chapters. The proofs are left as exercises.

Proposition 8.22. *In analogy to (7.14), for two discrete N-periodic functions f and g,*

$$\mathcal{F}_D(f \cdot g) = \frac{1}{N} (\mathcal{F}_D f) \bar{*} (\mathcal{F}_D g). \tag{8.25}$$

For a discrete function f, define the conjugate function $\bar{f}$ by setting $\bar{f}_k = \overline{f_k}$ for every k. In analogy to (5.10), we have the following fact.

Proposition 8.23. *For an N-periodic discrete function f,*

$$\left(\mathcal{F}_D \bar{f}\right)_j = \overline{(\mathcal{F}_D f)}_{-j} \tag{8.26}$$

for all j.

There is also a discrete version of the Rayleigh–Plancherel theorem 7.11:

Proposition 8.24. *For an N-periodic discrete function f,*

$$\sum_{n=0}^{N-1} |f_n|^2 = \frac{1}{N} \sum_{n=0}^{N-1} |(\mathcal{F}_D f)_n|^2. \tag{8.27}$$

8.7 Discrete back projection

In the continuous setting, the back projection is defined by

$$\mathcal{B}h(x, y) := \frac{1}{\pi} \int_{\theta=0}^{\pi} h(x\cos(\theta) + y\sin(\theta), \theta) \, d\theta. \tag{8.28}$$

Definition 8.25. In the discrete setting, the continuously variable angle θ is replaced by the discrete set of angles $\{k\pi/N : 0 \leq k \leq N-1\}$. So the value of $d\theta$ becomes π/N and the back-projection integral is replaced by the sum

$$\mathcal{B}_D h(x, y) = \left(\frac{1}{N}\right) \sum_{k=0}^{N-1} h(x\cos(k\pi/N) + y\sin(k\pi/N), k\pi/N). \tag{8.29}$$

Remark 8.26. We wish to apply formula (8.29) to $h = (\mathcal{F}_D^{-1}A)\bar{*}(\mathcal{R}_D f)$. The grid within which the final image is to be presented will be a rectangular array of pixels, located at a finite set of points $\{(x_m, y_n)\}$. We will compute the values $\mathcal{B}_D h(x_m, y_n)$, each of which represents a color or greyscale value to be assigned to the appropriate point in the grid. To do this, we require the values of $(\mathcal{F}_D^{-1}A)\bar{*}(\mathcal{R}_D f)$ at the corresponding points $\{(x_m \cos(k\pi/N) + y_n \sin(k\pi/N), k\pi/N)\}$. However, the X-ray scanner will give us samples of the Radon transform of f, and, hence, of $(\mathcal{F}_D^{-1}A)\bar{*}(\mathcal{R}_Df)$, only at the set of points $\{(j\tau, k\pi/N)\}$. These points are arranged in a polar grid and generally do not match up with the points needed.

To overcome this obstacle, observe that, for a given (x_m, y_n) and a given k, the number $x_m\cos(k\pi/N) + y_n\sin(k\pi/N)$ must lie in between some two consecutive integer multiples of τ. That is, there is some value $j_\sharp$ such that

$$j_\sharp\tau \leq x_m\cos(k\pi/N) + y_n\sin(k\pi/N) < (j_\sharp + 1)\tau.$$

Hence, we will *assign* a value for $(\mathcal{F}_D^{-1}A)\bar{*}(\mathcal{R}_Df)$ at $(x_m\cos(k\pi/N)+y_n\sin(k\pi/N), k\pi/N)$, based on the known values at the points $(j_\sharp\tau, k\pi/N)$ and $((j_\sharp + 1)\tau, k\pi/N)$ on either side. The process of assigning such values is called *interpolation*.

8.8 Interpolation

When we are given (or have computed) a discrete set of values $f_k = f(x_k)$ at a finite set of inputs $\{x_k\}$, the process of somehow assigning values $f(x)$ for inputs x between the distinct $\{x_k\}$ in order to create a continuous or, at least, piecewise continuous function defined on an interval is called *interpolation*. Exactly how the interpolated values are assigned depends on factors such as what additional properties (continuous, differentiable, infinitely differentiable, *et cetera*) the function is to have, the degree of computational difficulty incurred in assigning the new values, and more. Let us look at some interpolation schemes that are commonly used.

Nearest-neighbor. Given the values $\{f(x_k)\}$, nearest-neighbor interpolation assigns the value of $f(x)$, for any given x, to be the same as the value of f at the input x_k that is nearest to x. This creates a step function that steps up or down halfway between successive values of x_k. This is computationally simple, but the interpolated function is not continuous, and what to do at the halfway points between the x_k s is not clear.

Linear. With linear interpolation, we literally just connect the dots, thus creating a continuous function composed of line segments. Computationally, for x lying between x_k and x_{k+1}, we set

$$f(x) = \left(\frac{f(x_{k+1}) - f(x_k)}{x_{k+1} - x_k}\right) \cdot (x - x_k) + f(x_k). \tag{8.30}$$

This method is often used in medical imaging. It is computationally simple and produces a continuous function f. The interpolated function is usually not differentiable at the nodes.

Cubic spline. With cubic splines, each pair of successive points $(x_k, f(x_k))$ and $(x_{k+1}, f(x_{k+1}))$ is connected by part of a cubic curve, $y = ax^3 + bx^2 + cx + d$. We will design the pieces so that they join together smoothly, producing an overall curve with a continuous second-order derivative. This smoothness property often makes this method preferable to piecewise linear or nearest-neighbor interpolation. As we shall explore here, computing the coefficients of each cubic piece involves solving a system of linear equations. Thus, cubic splines are computationally more complicated than linear interpolation, but are still manageable. Splines are commonly used in a large variety of engineering applications, including medical imaging.

To see how this method works, suppose our sampled points are

$$\{(x_0, y_0), (x_1, y_1), \ldots, (x_n, y_n)\}, \text{ with } x_0 < x_1 < \ldots < x_n.$$

Our goal is to find n cubic curves, say $h_1, h_2, \ldots, h_n$ that we can piece together smoothly across our sample. Each cubic curve has four coefficients to be determined, so we will need a system of $4n$ equations in order to find them. We get $2n$, or half, of these equations from the requirement that the curves must fit the sample. That is, for each $k = 1, \ldots, n$, we need $h_k(x_{k-1}) = y_{k-1}$ and $h_k(x_k) = y_k$. Next, at each of the interior points $x_1, \ldots, x_{n-1}$ in the sample, we want the two cubic pieces that meet there to join together smoothly, meaning that the first- and second-order derivatives of the two pieces should agree at the transition. That is, for each $k = 1, \ldots, (n-1)$, we need $h_k'(x_k) = h_{k+1}'(x_k)$ and $h_k''(x_k) = h_{k+1}''(x_k)$. This produces $2(n-1)$ additional equations to the system, giving us $4n - 2$ equations so far. The remaining two equations are obtained by prescribing values for the initial slope of the first piece and the final slope of the last piece. That is, we assign values for $h_1'(x_0)$ and $h_n'(x_n)$. (For example, it may be convenient to assign the value 0 to these slopes.) Now we have the $4n$ equations we need.

Example 8.27. Suppose we wish to fit a cubic spline to the four sample points $(0, 1)$, $(1, 0.5)$, $(2, 4)$, and $(3, 3)$. There are three subintervals between the points, so we will need three cubic pieces. Here is one solution:

$$h(x) = \begin{cases} h_1(x) = \frac{41}{30}x^3 - \frac{28}{15}x + 1 & \text{if } 0 \leq x \leq 1, \\ h_2(x) = -\frac{17}{6}x^3 + \frac{63}{5}x^2 - \frac{217}{15}x + \frac{26}{5} & \text{if } 1 \leq x \leq 2, \\ h_3(x) = \frac{22}{15}x^3 - \frac{66}{5}x^2 + \frac{557}{15}x - \frac{146}{5} & \text{if } 2 \leq x \leq 3. \end{cases} \tag{8.31}$$

In this case, the values of $h_1'(0)$ and $h_3'(3)$ were unassigned, resulting in free variables in the linear system of equations.

Lagrange, or polynomial, interpolation. When $N + 1$ data points are known, then it is possible to fit a polynomial of degree N to the data. For instance, three noncollinear points determine a parabola. Generally, a polynomial of degree N has $N + 1$ coefficients. The $N + 1$ data points provide $N + 1$ equations that these coefficients must satisfy. A general formula, given values of $f(x_k)$ for $k = 1, \ldots, N + 1$, is

$$f(x) = \sum_{j=1}^{N+1} f(x_j) \cdot \frac{\prod_{k \neq j} (x - x_k)}{\prod_{k \neq j} (x_j - x_k)}. \tag{8.32}$$

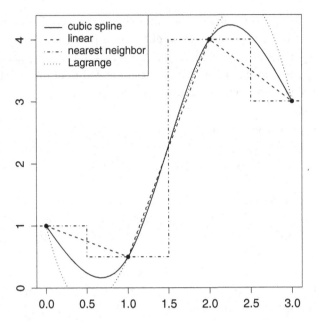

Fig. 8.3. Four methods for interpolating the sample points $(0, 1)$, $(1, 0.5)$, $(2, 4)$, and $(3, 3)$ are shown. The cubic spline has the formula from equation (8.31).

Notice that, if we take $x = x_n$ for some n, then the formula (8.32) yields $f(x) = f(x_n)$ as it should. So the formula agrees with the data. Polynomial interpolation can be problematic because we are using a single global polynomial to meet our needs. This is different from the other methods outlined here, in which piecewise functions are patched together to fit the sampled points. Thus, the polynomial may overshoot the sample points significantly while the piecewise functions would transition to another piece to avoid overshooting. Also, the degree of the polynomial increases with the size of the data set, so a large sample, typical in imaging and many other applications, requires a polynomial of high degree, while a cubic spline has degree 3. The relative merits of these interpolation methods can be glimpsed in Figure 8.3, which shows examples of nearest-neighbor, piecewise linear, cubic spline, and polynomial interpolation applied to a small data set.

Generalized interpolation. To see how the interpolation process can be generalized, take a closer look at nearest-neighbor interpolation. There, we start with a discrete function g, where $g(m)$ denotes the value of g at the sample point $m \cdot \tau$, and we want to construct an interpolated function $\mathcal{I}(g)$ using the nearest-neighbor method. For a given value x, the sample point $m \cdot \tau$ is the nearest neighbor to x exactly when $|x - m \cdot \tau| < \tau/2$, or, equivalently, when $|x/\tau - m| < 1/2$. It follows that

$$\mathcal{I}(g)(x) = \sum_m g(m) \cdot \sqcap_{1/2}\left(\frac{x}{\tau} - m\right), \quad \text{for all } x, \tag{8.33}$$

where, as usual,

$$\sqcap_{1/2}(x) = \begin{cases} 1 \text{ if } |x| < 1/2, \\ 0 \text{ if } |x| > 1/2. \end{cases}$$

(For $x = \pm 1/2$, make a slight modification by assigning the value $+1$ to one and 0 to the other, depending whether we want to consider $-1/2$ or $+1/2$ as closer to 0.) This approach offers a nice compact formula for nearest-neighbor interpolation.

Adopting a similar approach to linear interpolation, suppose that a given x satisfies

$$m_* \cdot \tau \leq x < (m_* + 1) \cdot \tau$$

for some integer m_*. Then

$$\left| \frac{x}{\tau} - m_* \right| \leq 1 \,,$$

$$\left| \frac{x}{\tau} - (m_* + 1) \right| \leq 1 \,,$$

and, for all integers m other than m_* and $(m_* + 1)$,

$$\left| \frac{x}{\tau} - m \right| > 1 \,.$$

Consider again the tent function $\bigwedge$, defined by

$$\bigwedge(x) = \begin{cases} 1 - |x| \text{ if } |x| \leq 1, \\ 0 \quad \text{ if } |x| > 1. \end{cases}$$

For a discrete function g, evaluated at the sample points $\{m \cdot \tau\}$, and the corresponding function $\mathcal{I}(g)$ obtained from g by linear interpolation, we get, for x satisfying $m_* \cdot \tau \leq x < (m_* + 1) \cdot \tau$,

$$\begin{aligned} \mathcal{I}(g)(x) &= \frac{g(m_* + 1) - g(m_*)}{\tau} \cdot (x - m_* \cdot \tau) + g(m_*) \\ &= (g(m_* + 1) - g(m_*)) \cdot \left(\frac{x}{\tau} - m_* \right) + g(m_*) \\ &= g(m_*) \left(1 - \left(\frac{x}{\tau} - m_* \right) \right) + g(m_* + 1) \left(\frac{x}{\tau} - m_* \right) \\ &= g(m_*) \left(1 - \left| \frac{x}{\tau} - m_* \right| \right) + g(m_* + 1) \left(1 - \left| \frac{x}{\tau} - (m_* + 1) \right| \right) \\ &= \sum_m g(m) \cdot \bigwedge \left(\frac{x}{\tau} - m \right) . \end{aligned} \tag{8.34}$$

Generalizing this approach, we can design an interpolation method like so.

Definition 8.28. For a selected weighting function W, satisfying the conditions below, the W-interpolation $\mathcal{I}_W(g)$ of a discrete function g is defined by

$$\mathcal{I}_W(g)(x) = \sum_m g(m) \cdot W\left(\frac{x}{\tau} - m\right) \text{ for } -\infty < x < \infty. \tag{8.35}$$

Of course, for this to be reasonable, the weighting function W should satisfy a few conditions. For instance, if g is real-valued, bounded, or even, then $\mathcal{I}_W(g)$ should be too, which means that W should be real-valued, bounded, and even. Also, at the sample points, we expect the interpolation to be exact. That is, for any integer k, we expect $\mathcal{I}_W(g)(k \cdot \tau) = g(k)$, which implies that $W(0) = 1$ and that $W(m) = 0$ for all integers $m \neq 0$. Lastly, for purposes of integration, it would be nice for W-interpolation to preserve areas in the sense that the integral of the W-interpolated function $\mathcal{I}_W(g)$ is actually *equal to* the approximation we get when we apply the trapezoidal rule to the sampled points $\{(m \cdot \tau, g(m))\}$. That is, we would like to have

$$\int_{-\infty}^{\infty} \mathcal{I}_W(g)(x)\, dx = \tau \cdot \sum_m g(m). \tag{8.36}$$

To see what this implies about W, observe that, for each integer m,

$$\int_{-\infty}^{\infty} W\left(\frac{x}{\tau} - m\right) dx = \tau \cdot \int_{-\infty}^{\infty} W(u - m)\, du \text{ where } u = x/\tau$$

$$= \tau \cdot \int_{-\infty}^{\infty} W(u)\, du.$$

In particular, the value of the integral is independent of m. From (8.35), we now compute

$$\int_{-\infty}^{\infty} \mathcal{I}_W(g)(x)\, dx = \int_{-\infty}^{\infty} \left\{ \sum_m g(m) \cdot W\left(\frac{x}{\tau} - m\right) \right\} dx$$

$$= \sum_m g(m) \cdot \int_{-\infty}^{\infty} W\left(\frac{x}{\tau} - m\right) dx$$

$$= \tau \cdot \int_{-\infty}^{\infty} W(u)\, du \cdot \sum_m g(m).$$

(The interchange of the summation and the integral is valid because we are summing over finitely many m.) Thus, for (8.36) to hold, we want W to satisfy

$$\int_{-\infty}^{\infty} W(u)\, du = 1.$$

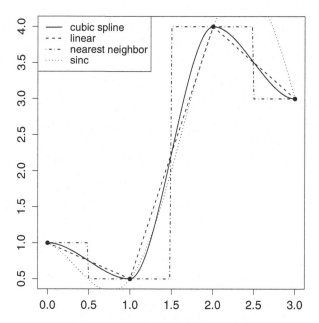

Fig. 8.4. Interpolating the sample points $(0, 1)$, $(1, 0.5)$, $(2, 4)$, and $(3, 3)$ using formula (8.35). The weight functions are: the cubic spline in (8.37), $\bigwedge$, $\sqcap_{1/2}$, and $\mathrm{sinc}(\pi x)$.

In addition to the functions $\sqcap_{1/2}$ and $\bigwedge$ considered above, the rescaled *sinc* function $x \mapsto \sin(\pi x)/(\pi x)$ also satisfies these conditions on the weighting function. We can implement a cubic spline interpolation with the weight function

$$W(x) = \begin{cases} -2x^2 - 3x^2 + 1 & \text{if } -1 \leq x \leq 0, \\ 2x^2 - 3x^2 + 1 & \text{if } 0 \leq x \leq 1, \\ 0 & \text{if } |x| > 1. \end{cases} \qquad (8.37)$$

This function defines a cubic spline joining the three points $(-1, 0)$, $(0, 1)$, and $(1, 0)$ with derivative equal to 0 at the endpoints. The interpolation formula (8.35) remodels it into a cubic spline that fits the data.

Example with R 8.29. Figure 8.4 was created by implementing formula (8.35) in *R*. For example, the following code can be used to carry out a cubic spline interpolation, with the weight function in (8.37). The lists `xdata` and `ydata` are the coordinates of the given data points, while `xval` is the list of points at which a function value is to be interpolated.

```
##cubic spline
Wspline=function(x){
(-2*x^3-3*x^2+1)*(-1<=x&x<=0)+(2*x^3-3*x^2+1)*(0<x&x<=1)}
xdata=0:3
ydata=c(1,0.5,4,3)
xval=.02*(0:150)#151 pts betw/ 0 and 3
#interpolate using spline window
```

```
y.y=double(length(xval))
for (i in 1:length(xval)){
y.y[i]=sum(ydata*Wspline((xval[i]-xdata)/xspace))}
```

Experiment with different sets of data points as well as different window functions W.

Interpolation and convolution. For a discrete function g and a weighting function W, let $\mathcal{I}_W(g)$ be as in (8.35). Suppose also that $g = \phi \bar{*} f$ for some discrete functions ϕ and f. That is, suppose that, for each m,

$$g(m) = \sum_k \phi(m-k) \cdot f(k) \, .$$

Then, for each x,

$$\mathcal{I}_W(g)(x) = \sum_m \left(\sum_k \phi(m-k) \cdot f(k) \right) \cdot W\left(\frac{x}{\tau} - m\right)$$

$$= \sum_k \left(\sum_m \phi(m-k) \cdot W\left(\frac{x}{\tau} - m\right) \right) \cdot f(k) \tag{8.38}$$

$$= \sum_k \left(\sum_m \phi(m-k) \cdot W\left(\frac{x-k\tau}{\tau} - (m-k)\right) \right) f(k).$$

We might mistake the sum $\sum_m \phi(m-k) \cdot W\left(((x-k\tau)/\tau) - (m-k)\right)$ in (8.38) for the interpolated function $\mathcal{I}_W(\phi)(x-k\tau)$. The discrete function ϕ is periodic after all, so shifting the summation from summing over m to summing over $(m-k)$ shouldn't matter. However, W is not periodic, so there is a glitch when $k = N-1$ for N-periodic functions. That's where ϕ wraps around but W does not. Nonetheless, it is *almost correct* to say that these two expressions are the same; and in practice, we can actually fix this glitch by using *zero padding*, as discussed following Proposition 8.17. So, from (8.38), we can write

$$\mathcal{I}_W(\phi \bar{*} f)(x) \approx \sum_k \mathcal{I}_W(\phi)(x-k\tau) \cdot f(k) \, . \tag{8.39}$$

The expression on the left in (8.39) represents an interpolation of the filtered form of f. On the right, the interpolation is brought inside and the expression has the form of a discrete convolution: a weighted average of the values $\{f(k)\}$, where the weights depend on the distance between x and the sampled points $\{k \cdot \tau\}$.

8.9   Discrete image reconstruction

We have now examined the discrete versions of all of the components of formula (8.2), and we are ready to realize our goal of reconstructing an attenuation-coefficient function f using a discrete set of samples of its Radon transform! In fact, there are two slightly different algorithms, depending on which side of the formula (8.39) we opt to use at the appropriate stage. Let us work our way through each algorithm step by step.

Example with R 8.30. Image Reconstruction Algorithm I. In our first implementation of (8.2), we apply interpolation to the convolution $(\mathcal{F}_D^{-1}A)\bar{*}(\mathcal{R}_D f)$, where A is the low-pass filter. Denoting this interpolated function by $\mathcal{I}$, we then approximate the value $f(x_m, y_n)$ at each point in the image grid by

$$f(x_m, y_n) \approx \left(\frac{1}{2}\right) \mathcal{B}_D \mathcal{I}(x_m, y_n)$$

$$= \left(\frac{1}{2N}\right) \sum_{k=0}^{N-1} \mathcal{I}\left(x_m \cos\left(\frac{k\pi}{N}\right) + y_n \sin\left(\frac{k\pi}{N}\right), \frac{k\pi}{N}\right). \tag{8.40}$$

As a test case, we will use the radially symmetric phantom shown on the left in Figure 8.5.

- We use R to compute the (discrete) Radon transform of this phantom, as in Example 2.13, in Chapter 2. (In a clinical setting, we would use actual X-ray data.) The data from the scan are recorded here in the vector `scan.1`.

```
##Phantom: a "bullseye"
P1=c(.75,.75,0,0,0,1)
P2=c(.5,.5,0,0,0,-.75)
P3=c(.25,.25,0,0,0,.25)
```

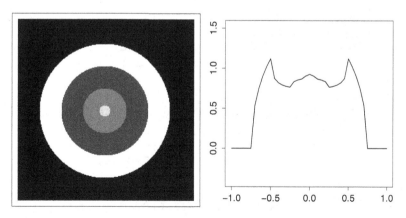

Fig. 8.5. A radially symmetric attenuation function and its Radon transform.

```
P4=c(.0625,.0625,0,0,0,.4)
P=matrix(c(P1,P2,P3,P4),byrow=T,ncol=6)
##Radon transform for elliptical regions
radon.mat=function(theta,t,E){
tmp=matrix(double(nrow(E)*length(theta)),nrow(E),length
   (theta))
for (i in 1:nrow(E)){
theta.1=theta-E[i,5]
t.1=(t-E[i,3]*cos(theta)-E[i,4]*sin(theta))/E[i,2]
v1=sin(theta.1)^2+(E[i,1]/E[i,2])^2*cos(theta.1)^2-t.1^2
v2=ifelse(sin(theta.1)^2+(E[i,1]/E[i,2])^2*cos(theta.1)^2
   -t.1^2>0,1,0)
v3=sqrt(v1*v2)
v4=sin(theta.1)^2+(E[i,1]/E[i,2])^2*cos(theta.1)^2
tmp[i,]=E[i,1]*E[i,6]*(v3/v4)}
radvec=colSums(tmp)
list(radvec=radvec)}
## apply Radon transform
scan.1=radon.mat(grid.theta,grid.t,P)$radvec
```

- The next step is to choose a low-pass filter A and compute its discrete inverse Fourier transform, $\mathcal{F}_D^{-1}A$. As discussed in Remark 8.17, when we interpret our low-pass filter as a $2L$-periodic discrete function that vanishes outside the interval $[-L, L]$, the effective sample spacing for $\mathcal{F}_D^{-1}A$ is given by $1/(2L)$. We then compute the discrete convolution $(\mathcal{F}_D^{-1}A)\bar{*}(\mathcal{R}_Df)$. The two discrete functions must have the same sample spacing, so we want to have $1/(2L) = \tau$. In practice, the value of τ is determined by the scanner, and, therefore, we set $L = 1/(2\tau)$ for the low-pass filter.

  For our test case, we use the Shepp–Logan filter and compute a separate discrete convolution for each angle. The output, called ffrad here, is a matrix with one row for each angle. (Due to the radial symmetry, these rows will all be the same.)

```
##DIFT of the Shepp-Logan filter:
L=(0.5)/tau #tau=X-ray spacing
IFSL=(4*L^2/pi^3)*(1/(1-4*((-1/tau):(1/tau))^2))#IFSL vals
#convolve scan.1 w/ IFSL #for each theta
#J=1+2/tau=no. of t vals
filter.rad=function(theta,f,g){
rad.fil=matrix(double(length(theta)*J),length(theta),J)
for (i in 1:length(theta)){
rad.fil[i,]=convolve(f[((i-1)*J+1):(i*J)],
rev(g),type="open")[(J-(1/tau)):(J+(1/tau))]}
list(rad.fil=rad.fil)}
#apply above procedure
ffrad=filter.rad(thetaval,scan.1,IFSL)$rad.fil
```

• Next, we select a method of interpolation. As we discussed in Remark 8.26, we will evaluate the discrete back projection only at a finite set of points $\{(x_m, y_n)\}$ that define the grid in which the final image is to be presented. We need interpolation in order to assign values to $(\mathcal{F}_D^{-1}A)\tilde{*}(\mathcal{R}_D f)$ at the points $\{(x_m \cos(k\pi/N) + y_n \sin(k\pi/N), k\pi/N)\}$.

We could execute a cubic spline interpolation as in Example 8.29. However, R, being a statistical tool, has built-in curve-fitting packages, including one for cubic splines. In this case, for each angle in the scan, a separate spline is computed to fit the data given by the corresponding row of the matrix of filtered X-ray data. (This is the matrix called `ffrad` in the previous step.) Then, for each point (x_m, y_n) in the image grid, we interpolate (or "predict" in the R procedure) values at the desired points. Basic code for this is given here. Figure 8.6 shows the resulting discrete function. (Compare this to the picture on the right in Figure 8.5.)

```
##load "splines" package: "library(splines)"
library(splines)
interp.mat=function(theta,tdata,M,x,y){
yy.mat=matrix(double(length(theta)*length(x)),length
    (theta),length(x))
for (i in 1:length(theta)){ydata=M[i,]
y.new=interpSpline(tdata,ydata)
t.new=cos(theta[i])*x+sin(theta[i])*y
yy.mat[i,]=predict(y.new,t.new)$y}
list(yy.mat=yy.mat)}
```

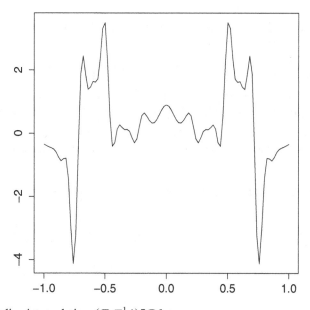

Fig. 8.6. The cubic spline interpolation $(\mathcal{F}_D^{-1}A)\tilde{*}\mathcal{R}f$.

```
## apply to ffrad on desired grid
ffrad.new=interp.mat(thetaval,tval,ffrad,grid.x,grid.y)
    $yy.mat
```

- Now that we have carried out the interpolation, we finish by applying the discrete back projection. For each point in the image grid, we compute the average, over all angles in the scan, of the corresponding interpolated values of the filtered X-ray data. In the previous step, ffrad.new is a matrix with one column of interpolated values for each grid point. Hence, the back projection amounts to computing the column averages of this matrix, like so.

```
#discrete back projection
backproj.discrete=function(M){
(1/nrow(M))*colSums(M)}
#apply to ffrad.new#then normalize colors to be betw/ 0
    and 1
colors.1=backproj.discrete(ffrad.new)
#final step: plot the result
colors.2=(colors.1-min(colors.1))/(max(colors.1)-min
    (colors.1))
#final step: plot the result
plot(grid.x,grid.y,pch=15,col=gray(colors.2),asp=1,
    xlab="",ylab="")
```

Figure 8.7 depicts two reconstructions of the test phantom. In both cases, we used a 100×100 grid in the square $\{(x, y) : |x| \le 1, |y| \le 1\}$ and sample spacing $\tau = 0.05$. The number of angle samples is 18 on the left and 60 for the picture on the right.

Example with R 8.31. Image Reconstruction Algorithm II. In our second image reconstruction algorithm, we use the approach indicated by the right-hand side of formula (8.39). Instead of interpolating the filtered Radon transform $(\mathcal{F}_D^{-1}A) \bar{*} (\mathcal{R}_D f)$, we first interpolate the filter itself and then form a weighted average of the sampled values of the Radon transform. That is, we replace each value of $\mathcal{I}$ in (8.40) by the weighted sum

$$\mathcal{W}(k) = \sum_j \mathcal{I}_{\mathcal{F}_D^{-1}A}\left(x_m \cos\left(\frac{k\pi}{N}\right) + y_n \sin\left(\frac{k\pi}{N}\right) - j\tau\right) \cdot \mathcal{R}_D f\left(j\tau, \frac{k\pi}{N}\right).$$

This leads to a slightly different approximation to the discrete filtered back projection given by

$$f(x_m, y_n) \approx \left(\frac{1}{2N}\right) \sum_{k=0}^{N-1} \mathcal{W}(k) . \tag{8.41}$$

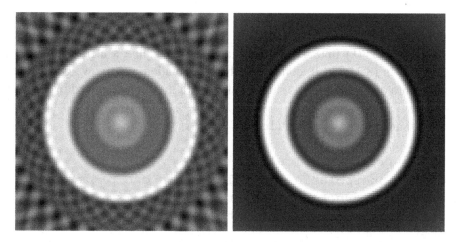

Fig. 8.7. The discrete filtered back-projection reconstruction of the bullseye. Algorithm (8.40) was used with sample spacing $\tau = 0.05$. The angle was sampled in increments of $\pi/18$ on the left and $\pi/60$ on the right. The discrete back projection was applied on a 100×100 grid.

This time, we will test our algorithm on the crescent-shaped phantom shown, along with its sinogram, in Figure 2.8, in Chapter 2.

- The phantom parameters are given below. We compute the (discrete) Radon transform as before, with scan.2 denoting the output vector.

```
##The "crescent" phantom
E1=c(.5,.5,0,0,0,1)
E2=c(.375,.375,.125,0,0,-.5)
E.mat=matrix(c(E1,E2),byrow=T,ncol=6)
## apply Radon transform as before
scan.2=radon.mat(grid.theta,grid.t,E.mat)$radvec
```

- For this example, we use the Ram–Lak low-pass filter, defined earlier. Again, the width of the window is $2L = 1/\tau$, and the effective sample-spacing for the discrete inverse Fourier transform is $1/(2L) = \tau$. We have

```
##Ram-Lak filter; inverse Fourier transform
L=(0.5)/tau
IFRL=function(n){
ifelse(n==0,(0.5)*L^2/pi,
((0.5)*L^2/pi)*(2*sin(pi*n)/(pi*n)-(sin(pi*n/2)/(pi*n/2)
   )^2))}
IFRL2=IFRL(tval/tau)#seq of IFRL vals
```

- The next step is where our two image reconstruction algorithms differ. This time, for each point (x, y) in the picture grid, and every point (t, θ) at which the Radon transform has been sampled, we first interpolate a value for the discrete inverse Fourier transform of the low-pass filter at $(x\cos(\theta) + y\sin(\theta) - t)$. Then we let t vary, and compute the weighted sum denoted by $\mathcal{W}(k)$ in (8.41). In this example, we use linear interpolation, calculating the values as in (8.34). In R, computing the interpolation and the weighted sum can be combined into one procedure, as shown below, with the output denoted by ffrad.3.

```
##use linear interpolation
tent1=function(x){
(1-abs(x))*(abs(x)<=1.0)}
#combine interpolation/convolution in one procedure
interp.algII=function(theta,t,v,x,y){
yy.mat=matrix(double(length(theta)*length(x)),length
  (theta),length(x))
for (i in 1:length(theta)){
ydata=v[((i-1)*J+1):(i*J)]#J=1+2/tau=no. of t vals
t.new=cos(theta[i])*x+sin(theta[i])*y
for (j in 1:length(x)){
filter.alt=double(length(t))
for (k in 1:length(t)){
filter.alt[k]=sum(IFRL2*tent1((t.new[j]-t[k]-t)/tau))}
yy.mat[i,j]=sum(ydata*filter.alt)}}
list(yy.mat=yy.mat)}
#apply to X-ray data (v=scan.2)
ffrad.3=interp.test3(thetaval,tval,scan.2,grid.x,grid.y)
  $yy.mat
```

- Finally, we apply the discrete back projection to ffrad3 by averaging the values in each column.

Figure 8.8 illustrates the resulting image reconstructions for two choices of angle increment: $\pi/60$ on the left and $\pi/36$ on the right. In both cases, we used the Ram–Lak low-pass filter, a sample spacing of $\tau = 0.02$ (so $L = 25$), and a 100×100 image grid.

Example 8.32. Image comparison. By altering the choices of algorithm, low-pass filter, interpolation method, and sample spacings, we can create a variety of reconstructions of the same phantom. Comparing the results helps us to assess how our choices affect the results. For example, the illustrations on the left sides of Figures 8.8 and 8.9 differ only in the choice of low-pass filter — Ram–Lak compared to Shepp–Logan. The picture on the right in Figure 8.9 depicts the difference between the two images. Locations where the two agree are shown as neutral grey; lighter or darker shades of grey indicate locations where the two reconstructions differ. For instance, a sort of halo effect can be seen at the outer boundary of the crescent.

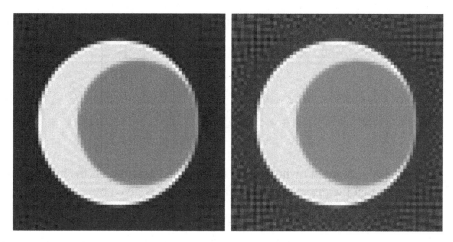

Fig. 8.8. The discrete filtered back-projection algorithm (8.41) is applied to a crescent-shaped phantom with sample spacing $\tau = 0.02$. The angle is sampled in increments of $\pi/60$ on the left and $\pi/36$ on the right.

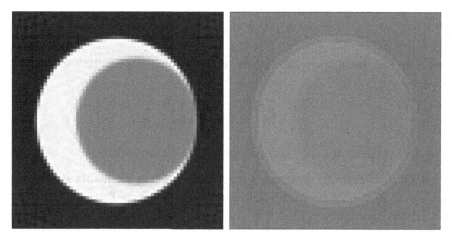

Fig. 8.9. On the left, algorithm (8.41) is applied to the crescent-shaped phantom using the Shepp–Logan filter with sample spacing $\tau = 0.02$ and angle increments of $\pi/60$. The figure on the right depicts the difference between this reconstruction and the one on the left in Figure 8.8, which used the Ram–Lak filter.

8.10 Matrix forms

For a discrete function $\mathbf{f} = \langle f_0, \ldots, f_{N-1} \rangle$ having period N, we have defined the discrete Fourier transform of $\mathbf{f}$ to be the discrete function $\mathbf{F} = \langle F_0, \ldots, F_{N-1} \rangle$, also having period N, satisfying

$$F_j = \sum_{k=0}^{N-1} f_k \, e^{-i2\pi kj/N} \text{ for } j = 0, 1, \ldots, (N-1).$$

Setting $w_N := e^{-i2\pi/N}$, we have $e^{-i2\pi kj/N} = (w_N)^{kj}$. Thus, in matrix form,

$$F_j = \begin{bmatrix} 1 & (w_N)^j & (w_N)^{2j} & \cdots & (w_N)^{(N-1)j} \end{bmatrix} \begin{bmatrix} f_0 \\ f_1 \\ f_2 \\ \vdots \\ f_{N-1} \end{bmatrix}. \tag{8.42}$$

Denote by $\mathbf{W}_N$ the $N \times N$ matrix whose entry in row j and column k is the number $(w_N)^{kj}$. It follows from (8.42) that the discrete Fourier transform of $\mathbf{f}$ is given by

$$\mathcal{F}_D \mathbf{f} = \mathbf{W}_N \mathbf{f}, \tag{8.43}$$

where $\mathbf{f}$ is viewed as a column vector in this context.

If we let $\overline{\mathbf{W}_N}$ denote the matrix obtained by taking the complex conjugates of the entries of $\mathbf{W}_N$, then it follows from Lemma 8.20 that $\overline{\mathbf{W}_N} \mathbf{W}_N = N \cdot I_N$. That is,

$$(\mathbf{W}_N)^{-1} = \frac{1}{N} \overline{\mathbf{W}_N},$$

from which we see that the inverse discrete Fourier transform can be expressed in matrix form as

$$\mathcal{F}_D^{-1} \mathbf{g} = \frac{1}{N} \overline{\mathbf{W}_N} \mathbf{g}, \tag{8.44}$$

where $\mathbf{g}$ is an N-periodic discrete function viewed as a column vector.

Example 8.33. This example illustrates the relation (8.24) in the matrix setting. With $N = 3$, we get $w_3 = e^{-i2\pi/3}$. For two discrete 3-periodic functions $\mathbf{f} = \langle f_0, f_1, f_2 \rangle$ and $\mathbf{g} = \langle g_0, g_1, g_2 \rangle$, the convolution is

$$\mathbf{f} \tilde{*} \mathbf{g} = \langle f_0 g_0 + f_1 g_2 + f_2 g_1, f_0 g_1 + f_1 g_0 + f_2 g_2, f_0 g_2 + f_1 g_1 + f_2 g_0 \rangle.$$

Hence,

$$\mathbf{W}_3(\mathbf{f} \tilde{*} \mathbf{g}) = \begin{bmatrix} 1 & 1 & 1 \\ 1 & w_3 & (w_3)^2 \\ 1 & (w_3)^2 & w_3 \end{bmatrix} \begin{bmatrix} f_0 g_0 + f_1 g_2 + f_2 g_1 \\ f_0 g_1 + f_1 g_0 + f_2 g_2 \\ f_0 g_2 + f_1 g_1 + f_2 g_0 \end{bmatrix}$$

$$= \begin{bmatrix} (f_0 + f_1 + f_2) \cdot (g_0 + g_1 + g_2) \\ (f_0 + w_3 f_1 + (w_3)^2 f_2) \cdot (g_0 + w_3 g_1 + (w_3)^2 g_2) \\ (f_0 + (w_3)^2 f_1 + w_3 f_2) \cdot (g_0 + (w_3)^2 g_1 + w_3 g_2) \end{bmatrix}$$

$$= (\mathbf{W}_3 \mathbf{f}) \cdot (\mathbf{W}_3 \mathbf{g}),$$

where the product in the last step is the entry-by-entry product of two vectors, each viewed as a discrete 3-periodic function.

8.11   FFT — the fast Fourier transform

For an N-periodic discrete function $\mathbf{f}$, the computation of the discrete Fourier transform of $\mathbf{f}$ requires N^2 multiplications, each of the form $f_k \cdot e^{-2\pi ikj/N}$ with $0 \leq k, j \leq N - 1$. For the large values of N encountered in medical imaging, this implies a significant amount of computational time. With the introduction, in [13], of the *fast Fourier transform*, Cooley and Tukey showed that the computation time can be reduced substantially — by a factor of $\log(N)/N$ — if N is a power of 2.

For starters, suppose that N is an even number, say $N = 2 \cdot M$. Then the Nth roots of unity can be divided into two sets. Those of the form $e^{-2\pi i(2k)j/N} = e^{-2\pi ikj/M}$, for $0 \leq k \leq (M-1)$, are also M^{th} roots of unity. The rest have the form $e^{-2\pi i(2k+1)j/N} = e^{-2\pi ij/N} \cdot e^{-2\pi ikj/M}$, for $0 \leq k \leq (M - 1)$. Thus, for each j between 0 and $(N - 1)$, the corresponding component of the discrete Fourier transform of $\mathbf{f}$ can be expressed as

$$(\mathcal{F}_D\mathbf{f})_j = \sum_{k=0}^{M-1} f_{2k} \cdot e^{-2\pi ikj/M} + \left(e^{-2\pi i/N}\right)^j \cdot \sum_{k=0}^{M-1} f_{2k+1} \cdot e^{-2\pi ikj/M}. \tag{8.45}$$

Moreover, for $0 \leq k \leq (M - 1)$ and $M \leq j \leq (N - 1)$, we get

$$e^{-2\pi ikj/M} = e^{-2\pi ik(j-M)/M} \cdot e^{-2\pi ikM/M} = e^{-2\pi ik(j-M)/M}. \tag{8.46}$$

In other words, for $M \leq j \leq (N - 1)$, we may replace j with $(j - M)$ in the sums on the right-hand side of (8.45). Also, $\left(e^{-2\pi i/N}\right)^j = -\left(e^{-2\pi i/N}\right)^{j-M}$. So now we can express the discrete Fourier transform of $\mathbf{f}$ in an even simpler way. Namely, for $0 \leq j \leq (M-1)$, we have

$$(\mathcal{F}_D\mathbf{f})_j = \sum_{k=0}^{M-1} f_{2k} \cdot e^{-2\pi ikj/M} + \left(e^{-2\pi i/N}\right)^j \cdot \sum_{k=0}^{M-1} f_{2k+1} \cdot e^{-2\pi ikj/M} \tag{8.47}$$

and

$$(\mathcal{F}_D\mathbf{f})_{j+M} = \sum_{k=0}^{M-1} f_{2k} \cdot e^{-2\pi ikj/M} - \left(e^{-2\pi i/N}\right)^j \cdot \sum_{k=0}^{M-1} f_{2k+1} \cdot e^{-2\pi ikj/M}. \tag{8.48}$$

The beauty of this is that, for $N = 2M$, we have now represented the discrete Fourier transform of the N-periodic discrete function $\mathbf{f}$ in terms of the discrete Fourier transforms of *two* M-periodic discrete functions $\mathbf{f}^0 = \{f_{2k} : 0 \leq k \leq M - 1\}$ and $\mathbf{f}^1 = \{f_{2k+1} : 0 \leq k \leq M - 1\}$. In symbols,

$$(\mathcal{F}_D\mathbf{f})_j = \left(\mathcal{F}_D\mathbf{f}^0\right)_j + \left(e^{-2\pi i/N}\right)^j \cdot \left(\mathcal{F}_D\mathbf{f}^1\right)_j \tag{8.49}$$

and

$$\left(\mathcal{F}_D\mathbf{f}\right)_{j+M} = \left(\mathcal{F}_D\mathbf{f}^0\right)_j - \left(e^{-2\pi i/N}\right)^j \cdot \left(\mathcal{F}_D\mathbf{f}^1\right)_j, \qquad (8.50)$$

for $0 \leq j \leq (M-1)$. Assuming that $\left(\mathcal{F}_D\mathbf{f}^0\right)$ and $\left(\mathcal{F}_D\mathbf{f}^1\right)$ have already been computed, then only two multiplications are required to compute each component of $(\mathcal{F}_D\mathbf{f})$, for a total of $2N$ multiplications. (For each component, there is one multiplication by the factor 1 and another by the factor $\pm e^{-2\pi ij/N}$.)

Now, if $M = N/2$ also happens to be an even number, then we can apply the same reasoning to split each of the M-periodic discrete functions $\mathbf{f}^0$ and $\mathbf{f}^1$ into two $M/2$-periodic functions. The discrete Fourier transforms of $\mathbf{f}^0$ and $\mathbf{f}^1$ can be computed from those of the corresponding pair using $2M$ multiplications each, for a total of $2 \cdot 2M = 2N$ multiplications. We now see that, if $N = 2^p$ is a power of 2, then we can continue this process of splitting discrete functions into pairs of discrete functions, halving the period at each stage, until we are left with 2^p separate 1-periodic discrete functions — the individual components of the original function $\mathbf{f}$. Each of these components is equal to its own discrete Fourier transform (apply the definition (8.19)), so we can start from there, forming pairs, computing discrete Fourier transforms, and building back up to $\mathbf{f}$. Each stage in the process will require $2N$ multiplications, and there are p stages until we reach the discrete Fourier transform of $\mathbf{f}$. The total number of multiplications required is, therefore, $2Np = 2N\log_2(N)$, which, for large values of N, compares favorably to the N^2 products required if (8.19) is used. For example, if $N = 2^{16} = 65536$, then $2N\log_2(N)$ is less than 0.05% of N^2. Moreover, many of the multiplications involved are actually just multiplication by the factor 1; so the savings in computation time may be even greater than it initially appears. This method is called the *fast Fourier transform*.

Some care must be taken in how the individual components of $\mathbf{f}$ are paired up if we are eventually to arrive at the functions $\mathbf{f}^0$ and $\mathbf{f}^1$ and then, finally, at $\mathbf{f}$. In the first stage, form separate lists of the components with even subscripts (f_0, f_2, and so on) and those with odd subscripts (f_1, f_3, etc.). Then pair the components in the first half of each list with those in the second half of the list. Thus, f_0 is paired with $f_{N/2}$, f_2 with $f_{N/2+2}$, and so on up to the pair $f_{N/2-2}$ and f_{N-2}. Similarly, f_1 is paired with $f_{N/2+1}$, f_3 with $f_{N/2+3}$, up to the pair $f_{N/2-1}$ and f_{N-1}. The discrete Fourier transform of each pair is computed from the transforms of its two components. For the next stage, the pairs in the even list are paired up according to the same scheme: those in the first half of the list are paired with those in the second half. In the same way, the pairs in the first half of the odd list are matched up with the pairs in the second half of the odd list. This pattern then replicates from stage to stage until, in the penultimate stage, all of the components with even subscripts are combined in the same $N/2$-periodic discrete function, and those with odd subscripts make up another discrete function. In the final stage, the evens and odds are reunited at last.

Example 8.34. Fast Fourier transform for an 8-periodic discrete function. Let $\mathbf{f}$ be an 8-periodic discrete function. To compute the discrete Fourier transform of $\mathbf{f}$ via the fast Fourier transform algorithm, begin with the separate components of $\mathbf{f}$ and pair them up as (f_0, f_4), (f_2, f_6), (f_1, f_5), and (f_3, f_7). The discrete Fourier transforms of these pairs are, respectively,

$$\{f_0 + f_4, f_0 - f_4\}, \ \{f_2 + f_6, f_2 - f_6\}, \ \{f_1 + f_5, f_1 - f_5\},$$
$$\text{and } \{f_3 + f_7, f_3 - f_7\}.$$

For the next stage, merge pairs of 2-periodic functions to form two 4-periodic functions: $\{(f_0, f_4), (f_2, f_6)\}$ and $\{(f_1, f_5), (f_3, f_7)\}$. By (8.49) and (8.50), the discrete transforms of these pairs are, respectively,

$$\{(f_0 + f_4) + (f_2 + f_6), \ (f_0 - f_4) - i \cdot (f_2 - f_6),$$
$$(f_0 + f_4) - (f_2 + f_6), \ (f_0 - f_4) + i \cdot (f_2 - f_6)\}$$

and

$$\{(f_1 + f_5) + (f_3 + f_7), \ (f_1 - f_5) - i \cdot (f_3 - f_7),$$
$$(f_1 + f_5) - (f_3 + f_7), \ (f_1 - f_5) + i \cdot (f_3 - f_7)\}.$$

Finally, combine the two 4-periodic functions into the single 8-periodic function $\mathbf{f} = \{[(f_0, f_4), (f_2, f_6)], [(f_1, f_5), (f_3, f_7)]\}$. Again following from (8.49) and (8.50), the discrete transform is

$$\mathcal{F}_D \mathbf{f} = \{\ [(f_0 + f_4) + (f_2 + f_6)] + [(f_1 + f_5) + (f_3 + f_7)],$$
$$[(f_0 - f_4) - i \cdot (f_2 - f_6)] + e^{-\pi i/4}\,[(f_1 - f_5) - i \cdot (f_3 - f_7)],$$
$$[(f_0 + f_4) - (f_2 + f_6)] - i[(f_1 + f_5) - (f_3 + f_7)],$$
$$[(f_0 - f_4) + i \cdot (f_2 - f_6)] + e^{-3\pi i/4}\,[(f_1 - f_5) + i \cdot (f_3 - f_7)],$$
$$\{\ [(f_0 + f_4) + (f_2 + f_6)] - [(f_1 + f_5) + (f_3 + f_7)],$$
$$[(f_0 - f_4) - i \cdot (f_2 - f_6)] - e^{-\pi i/4}\,[(f_1 - f_5) - i \cdot (f_3 - f_7)],$$
$$[(f_0 + f_4) - (f_2 + f_6)] + i[(f_1 + f_5) - (f_3 + f_7)],$$
$$[(f_0 - f_4) + i \cdot (f_2 - f_6)] - e^{-3\pi i/4}\,[(f_1 - f_5) + i \cdot (f_3 - f_7)]\}.$$

This agrees with (8.19), and if one counts every instance of a coefficient other than 1, the total number of multiplications involved is only about half of $8^2 = 64$ (though, admittedly, $N = 8$ is too small for there to be much of a savings here).

If this is applied to the 8-periodic discrete function with $f_k = \cos(\pi k/2)$ for $0 \le k \le 7$, the resulting discrete Fourier transform is

$$\mathcal{F}_D \mathbf{f} = \{0, 0, 4, 0, 0, 0, 4, 0\}.$$

Thus, the amplitude of the *cosine* wave is evenly divided between two opposite frequencies. This corresponds to the continuous setting in which the continuous Fourier transform of the *cosine* function consists of two impulses at opposite frequencies.

The fast Fourier transform has a matrix implementation as well. This amounts to factoring the matrix $\mathbf{W}_N$ in (8.43) in the case where $N = 2^p$. As in (8.43), an N-periodic discrete function $\mathbf{f}$ is viewed as a column vector,

$$
\mathbf{f} = \begin{bmatrix} f_0 \\ f_1 \\ f_2 \\ \vdots \\ f_{N-1} \end{bmatrix}.
$$

The initial step of rearranging the components of $\mathbf{f}$ for the first round of pairing is implemented using a matrix obtained by rearranging the rows of the $N \times N$ identity matrix. Specifically, if $\mathbf{e}_k$ denotes the kth row of the identity matrix, then let E_N denote the matrix

$$
E_N := \begin{bmatrix} \mathbf{e}_0 \\ \mathbf{e}_{N/2} \\ \mathbf{e}_2 \\ \mathbf{e}_{N/2+2} \\ \vdots \\ \mathbf{e}_{N/2-2} \\ \mathbf{e}_{N-2} \\ \mathbf{e}_1 \\ \mathbf{e}_{N/2+1} \\ \vdots \\ \mathbf{e}_{N/2-1} \\ \mathbf{e}_{N-1} \end{bmatrix}.
$$

Then $E_N \mathbf{f}$ achieves the desired reordering of the components of $\mathbf{f}$.

As in (8.43), let $w_N = e^{-2\pi i/N}$ and, for each integer k with $1 \le k \le p$, let R_k be the $2^{k-1} \times 2^{k-1}$ diagonal matrix with entries $\left((w_N)^{2^{p-k}} \right)^j$ in the jth diagonal position, for $0 \le j \le 2^{k-1} - 1$. Let I denote the identity matrix (in this case, of dimensions $2^{k-1} \times 2^{k-1}$) and define a $2^k \times 2^k$ matrix B_k by

$$
B_k := \left[\begin{array}{c|c} I & R_k \\ \hline I & -R_k \end{array} \right]. \tag{8.51}
$$

Multiplication by B_k computes the discrete Fourier transform of a 2^k-periodic discrete function from the transforms of a pair of 2^{k-1}-periodic functions. Thus, defining a $2^p \times 2^p$ block-diagonal matrix T_k by arranging 2^{p-k} copies of B_k along the diagonal, it follows that multiplication by T_k computes the discrete transforms of 2^{p-k} different 2^k-periodic discrete functions. This corresponds to the kth stage of the fast Fourier transform algorithm. The end result of this algorithm is therefore described by the product

$$
\mathcal{F}_D \mathbf{f} = T_p \cdot T_{p-1} \cdots T_1 \cdot E_N \mathbf{f}. \tag{8.52}
$$

For example, when $N = 4$, we get

$$E_4 = \begin{bmatrix} 1 & 0 & 0 & 0 \\ 0 & 0 & 1 & 0 \\ 0 & 1 & 0 & 0 \\ 0 & 0 & 0 & 1 \end{bmatrix}, \quad T_1 = \begin{bmatrix} 1 & 1 & 0 & 0 \\ 1 & -1 & 0 & 0 \\ 0 & 0 & 1 & 1 \\ 0 & 0 & 1 & -1 \end{bmatrix},$$

and

$$T_2 = \begin{bmatrix} 1 & 0 & 1 & 0 \\ 0 & 1 & 0 & -i \\ 1 & 0 & -1 & 0 \\ 0 & 1 & 0 & i \end{bmatrix}.$$

With $\mathbf{f} = \{f_0, f_1, f_2, f_3\}$, we have

$$\mathcal{F}_D \mathbf{f} = T_2 \cdot T_1 \cdot E_4 \mathbf{f}$$

$$= \begin{bmatrix} 1 & 0 & 1 & 0 \\ 0 & 1 & 0 & -i \\ 1 & 0 & -1 & 0 \\ 0 & 1 & 0 & i \end{bmatrix} \begin{bmatrix} 1 & 1 & 0 & 0 \\ 1 & -1 & 0 & 0 \\ 0 & 0 & 1 & 1 \\ 0 & 0 & 1 & -1 \end{bmatrix} \begin{bmatrix} 1 & 0 & 0 & 0 \\ 0 & 0 & 1 & 0 \\ 0 & 1 & 0 & 0 \\ 0 & 0 & 0 & 1 \end{bmatrix} \begin{bmatrix} f_0 \\ f_1 \\ f_2 \\ f_3 \end{bmatrix}.$$

Each of the matrices T_k has the property that there are only two nonzero entries in each row and each column. Thus, the matrix product in (8.52) requires only $2N$ multiplications for each factor. There are p factors in all, not counting E_N (which requires no multiplications), for a total of $2Np = 2N \log_2(N)$ multiplications, as we found before. Again, many of these multiplications involve the factor 1.

8.12 Fan beam geometry

In order to implement the discrete filtered back-projection formulas (8.2) and (8.40), it is necessary to know the values of $\mathcal{R}f(t, \theta)$ for a variety of choices of t for each of the selected angles θ. Conceptually, we have envisioned a scanning machine that sends out a set of parallel X-ray beams at each selected angle and records the corresponding values of the Radon transform. Such a machine would have to have a strip of distinct transmitters spaced at an appropriate sample spacing and able to rotate as a single unit during the scanning process. Each setting would correspond to a particular value of $\theta = k\pi/N$, and, once the readings had been taken, the corresponding summand in (8.40) could be calculated. This corresponds to the parallel beam geometry that has been the basis of our analysis all along.

In practice, however, it is easier to design a machine that has a single X-ray beam transmitter that emits a fan of beams. An arc of detectors on the other side measures the

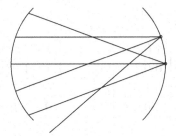

Fig. 8.10. Different fans yield parallel beams.

values of the Radon transform along the lines corresponding to the beams in the fan. The trouble is that each transmission includes beams at a variety of values of θ. Observe, though, that if two beams in the fan make an angle of ϕ with each other when they are emitted, then, when the transmitter itself has been rotated by the same angle ϕ and the two beams are emitted again, one of the new beams will be parallel to one of the beams from the previous transmission. (See Figure 8.10 for an illustration of this.) In other words, once the scanning process has been completed, it is possible to reorganize the fan beam data into an equivalent collection of parallel beam data. The image reconstruction algorithm can then be applied to this reorganized data to produce an image. This approach is called the *fan beam geometry*.

Rather than go into more detail here, we leave an examination of the fan beam geometry as a topic for further study. Other scanning geometries that have been developed for use in later generation scanning machines include the spiral beam and cone beam geometries, both of which facilitate the collection of data for more than one slice at the same time. The overarching goal in the design of new geometries is to lessen the radiation exposure of the patient by increasing the efficiency of the collection of the X-ray data. More information can be found in the article [52] and the books [12] and [32].

8.13 Exercises

1. Consider the low-pass cosine filter (7.29):

$$A(\omega) = |\omega| \cdot \cos(\pi\omega/(2L)) \cdot \sqcap_L(\omega)$$

$$= \begin{cases} |\omega| \cos(\pi\omega/(2L)) & \text{if } |\omega| \leq L \\ 0 & \text{if } |\omega| > L \end{cases}.$$

Following the format used for the Shepp–Logan and Ram–Lak filters in Section 8.3,

(a) compute the inverse Fourier transform $\mathcal{F}^{-1}A$, and

(b) show that

$$(\mathcal{F}^{-1}A)(\pi n/L) = \left(\frac{2 \cdot L^2}{\pi^3}\right) \cdot \left(\frac{\pi \cdot \cos(\pi n)}{(1 - 4n^2)} - \frac{2 \cdot (1 + 4n^2)}{(1 - 4n^2)^2}\right)$$

for all integers n.

(c) Use R, as in example 8.5, to plot the filter A and the sampled points of its inverse Fourier transform.

2. Prove Proposition 8.9: For discrete functions f, g, and h, and any constant α,

(a) $f \bar{*} g = g \bar{*} f$,
(b) $f \bar{*} (g + h) = f \bar{*} g + f \bar{*} h$, and
(c) $f \bar{*} (\alpha g) = \alpha (f \bar{*} g)$.

(Assume that all of the sums converge.)

3. Prove Proposition 8.22: For two discrete N-periodic functions f and g,

$$\mathcal{F}_D(f \cdot g) = \frac{1}{N} (\mathcal{F}_D f) \bar{*} (\mathcal{F}_D g) . \tag{8.53}$$

Note that this is analogous to (7.14).

4. For a discrete function f, define the conjugate function $\bar{f}$ by setting $\bar{f}_k = \overline{f_k}$ for every k. In analogy to (5.10), prove Proposition 8.23:

$$\left(\mathcal{F}_D \bar{f}\right)_j = \overline{(\mathcal{F}_D f)}_{-j} \tag{8.54}$$

for all j. (Note that $(\mathcal{F}_D f)_{-j} = (\mathcal{F}_D f)_{N-j}$ by periodicity.)

5. Prove Proposition 8.24, the discrete Rayleigh–Plancherel theorem: For an N-periodic discrete function f,

$$\sum_{n=0}^{N-1} |f_n|^2 = \frac{1}{N} \sum_{n=0}^{N-1} |(\mathcal{F}_D f)_n|^2 . \tag{8.55}$$

6. Prove the identity (8.20):

$$1/2 + \cos(\theta) + \cos(2\theta) + \cdots + \cos(M\theta) = \frac{\sin((M + 1/2)\theta)}{2 \cdot \sin(\theta/2)},$$

for all natural numbers M and all real θ. (The function $D_M(\theta) = \frac{\sin((M+1/2)\theta)}{\sin(\theta/2)}$ is called the *Dirichlet kernel*, after Peter Gustav Lejeune Dirichlet (1805–1859). The convolution of D_M with a function f having period 2π is equal to the Mth-degree Fourier series approximation to f.)

7. On the interval $0 \le x \le 1$, write down a formula for the piecewise linear function F determined by the values $F(0) = 0.5$, $F(1/3) = 0.3$, $F(2/3) = 0.6$, and $F(1) = 0.5$. (The formula should consist of three line segments.) Then use this formula to compute the values $F(0.2)$ and $F(0.7)$.

8. Recall the formula (8.32) for Lagrange interpolation of a function f using $N + 1$ data points $(x_1, f(x_1)), \ldots, (x_{N+1}, f(x_{N+1}))$:

$$f(x) = \sum_{j=1}^{N+1} f(x_j) \cdot \frac{\prod_{k \ne j} (x - x_k)}{\prod_{k \ne j} (x_j - x_k)}.$$

   Verify that, if $x = x_n$ for some n between 1 and $N + 1$, then the formula yields $f(x) = f(x_n)$. (Thus, the formula agrees with the data.)

9. (a) Verify that the cubic spline given in equation (8.31) passes through the points $(0, 1)$, $(1, 0.5)$, $(2, 4)$, and $(3, 3)$.
   (b) Verify that the cubic pieces on adjacent subintervals have the same first- and second-order derivatives at the transition.
   (c) Evaluate $h_1'(0)$ and $h_3'(3)$.
   (d) Compute a cubic spline that passes through the same sample points but has derivative 0 at each end point.
   (e) Use a graphing device to compare the graphs of the spline in equation (8.31) and the spline just computed in part (d).

10. Use formula (8.32) to compute the formula for the polynomial that interpolates the sample points $(0, 1)$, $(1, 0.5)$, $(2, 4)$, and $(3, 3)$. Compare the graph of this polynomial to those of the cubic splines from exercise 9.

11. Consider the sampled data $(0, 1)$, $(1, 0.5)$, $(2, 4)$, and $(3, 3)$. We may view this as corresponding to a discrete function g where $g(0) = 1$, $g(1) = 0.5$, $g(2) = 4$, and $g(3) = 3$. Use formula (8.35) to compute the interpolated values $\mathcal{I}_W(g)(0.6)$, $\mathcal{I}_W(g)(1.2)$, and $\mathcal{I}_W(g)(2.4)$ for each of the following weight functions. (Note that the sample spacing is $\tau = 1$.)

   (a) $W = \sqcap_{1/2}$;
   (b) $W = \wedge$;
   (c) $W : x \mapsto \sin(\pi x)/(\pi x)$;
   (d) W as in (8.37).

12. Apply the work in Example 8.34 to the 8-periodic discrete function with $f_k = \cos(\pi k/2)$ for $0 \le k \le 7$. Verify that the resulting discrete Fourier transform is

$$\mathcal{F}_D \mathbf{f} = \{0, 0, 4, 0, 0, 0, 4, 0\}.$$

   As observed above, this divides the amplitude of the *cosine* wave among two opposite frequencies, analogous to the continuous Fourier transform of the *cosine* function.

9

Algebraic Reconstruction Techniques

9.1 Introduction

To this point, we have studied how Fourier transform methods are used in image reconstruction. This is the approach taken in the seminal work of Cormack [14] and used in the algorithms of today's CT scan machines. However, the first CT scanner, designed in the late 1960s, by Godfrey Hounsfield, used an approach grounded in linear algebra and matrix theory to generate an image from the machine readings. Algorithms that adopt this point of view are known as *algebraic reconstruction techniques*, or ART, for short. In this chapter, we look at a few basic mathematical elements of ART.

Where the Fourier transform methods begin with a continuous theory — the filtered back-projection formula of Theorem 6.2 — which is then modeled using discrete methods, ART treats the problem of image reconstruction as a discrete problem from the start. Any image that we produce will be constructed inside a rectangular grid of picture elements, or pixels. The number of pixels in a given image may be large, but it is nonetheless finite, typically on the order of 10^5. For example, there are 65536 pixels in a 256-by-256 grid. To form an image, a specific color value is assigned to each pixel. For instance, the color value assigned to a given pixel might be a *greyscale* value, a number between 0 (= black) and 1 (= white), that represents the density or attenuation coefficient of the matter in the sample at the location of the given pixel. ART techniques use a system of constraints derived from the machine readings to compute these color values.

So, suppose an image is to be constructed in a K-by-K grid of pixels. Each pixel is really a small square in the plane. For convenience, number the pixels like so: 1 through K from left to right across the top row; $K + 1$ through $2K$ across the second row; and so on until, in the bottom row, we find pixels numbered $(K - 1)K + 1$ through K^2. Next, define the *pixel basis functions* $b_1, \ldots, b_{K^2}$ by

Electronic supplementary material The online version of this chapter (doi: 10.1007/978-3-319-22665-1_9) contains supplementary material, which is available to authorized users.

T.G. Feeman, *The Mathematics of Medical Imaging*, Springer Undergraduate Texts in Mathematics and Technology, DOI 10.1007/978-3-319-22665-1_9

$$b_k(x, y) = \begin{cases} 1 & \text{if } (x, y) \text{ lies inside pixel number } k, \\ 0 & \text{if } (x, y) \text{ does not lie inside pixel number } k \end{cases} \tag{9.1}$$

for $k = 1, 2, \ldots, K^2$ and points (x, y) in the plane. If we assign the color value x_k to the kth pixel, then the resulting image will be represented by the function

$$\widetilde{f}(x, y) = \sum_{k=1}^{K^2} x_k \cdot b_k(x, y) \tag{9.2}$$

for each point (x, y) lying inside the overall region covered by the grid. Applying the Radon transform $\mathcal{R}$ to both sides of this equation, and using the linearity of $\mathcal{R}$, we get, for each choice of t and θ,

$$\mathcal{R}\widetilde{f}(t, \theta) = \sum_{k=1}^{K^2} x_k \cdot \mathcal{R}b_k(t, \theta). \tag{9.3}$$

In practice, the X-ray machine gives us the values of $\mathcal{R}\widetilde{f}(t, \theta)$ for some finite set of lines $\ell_{t, \theta}$. For convenience, let's say these known values correspond to (t_1, θ_1), (t_2, θ_2), ..., (t_J, θ_J) for some positive integer J. Then,

$$\text{let } p_j = \mathcal{R}\widetilde{f}(t_j, \theta_j), \text{ for } j = 1, 2, \ldots, J.$$

The equation (9.3) can now be written as a system of equations

$$p_j = \sum_{k=1}^{K^2} x_k \cdot \mathcal{R}b_k(t_j, \theta_j) \text{ for } j = 1, \ldots, J. \tag{9.4}$$

Our next observation is that, since the pixel basis function b_k has the value 1 on its pixel and 0 elsewhere, the value of the integral $\mathcal{R}b_k(t_j, \theta_j)$ is equal to the *length of the intersection* of the line ℓ_{t_j, θ_j} with pixel number k. In principle, these values are easy to compute. (*Caveat:* If we allow finite-width X-ray beams, rather than zero-width, then this computation becomes more complicated.) So, let's denote by r_{jk} the length of the intersection of the line ℓ_{t_j, θ_j} with pixel number k; that is,

$$\text{let } r_{jk} = \mathcal{R}b_k(t_j, \theta_j) \text{ for } j = 1, \ldots, J \text{ and } k = 1, \ldots, K^2. \tag{9.5}$$

With this notation, the system (9.4) can be written as

$$p_j = \sum_{k=1}^{K^2} x_k \cdot r_{jk} \text{ for } j = 1, \ldots, J. \tag{9.6}$$

This is a system of J linear equations in K^2 unknowns $(x_1, \ldots, x_{K^2})$. Typically, both J and K^2 are on the order of 10^5, so the system is large. However, any particular line ℓ_{t_j, θ_j} passes through relatively few of the pixels in the grid, on the order of K out of K^2 total pixels. Thus, most of the values r_{jk} are equal to 0, meaning that the system (9.6) is large but *sparse*. With typical values of J and K, only about one percent of the entries in the coefficient matrix of the system are nonzero.

The system (9.6) can also be expressed in matrix form $A\mathbf{x} = \mathbf{p}$ by taking A to be the $J \times K^2$ matrix whose jth row is the (row) vector $\mathbf{r}_j = [r_{j1}, \ldots, r_{jK^2}]$, $\mathbf{x}$ to be the (column) vector in $\mathbb{R}^{K^2}$ with kth entry x_k, and $\mathbf{p}$ to be the (column) vector in $\mathbb{R}^J$ with jth coordinate p_j.

Some computational concerns arise from this approach to the image reconstruction problem. For one thing, the system of equations we have to solve is *large* — typically on the order of 10^5 equations. Each sampling of the Radon transform produces an equation in the system while each pixel corresponds to an unknown, the color value for that pixel. If the system of equations is overdetermined, with more equations than unknowns, then the system likely does not have an exact solution. If the system is underdetermined, with more unknowns than equations, then there may be infinitely many solutions, only one of which could possibly be the correct solution. A typical scan might include 200 X-ray measurements at each of 180 different directions, for a total of 36000 equations in the system. A grid of 160×160 pixels gives 25600 unknowns and an overdetermined system. To get an image with higher resolution, though, we may want to use a grid of 256×256 pixels, or 65536 unknowns. This results in a system that is heavily underdetermined, so the iterative algorithms discussed below are ineffective. For this reason, among others, iterative algorithms are not widely used in commercial CT machines. In any case, due to errors in measurement in sampling the Radon transform, the equations are only estimates to begin with. So, again, the system is not likely to have an exact solution. The fact that the coefficient matrix is *sparse*, with only a small proportion of nonzero entries, also has a direct effect on the computational complexity.

We now look at several different methods for arriving at an approximate solution to a system of linear equations. The first is an iterative approach called Kaczmarz's method, while the others are based on least squares approximation.

9.2 Kaczmarz's method

Kaczmarz's method is an iterative procedure, or algorithm, for approximating a solution to a linear system $A\mathbf{x} = \mathbf{p}$. If we denote by $\mathbf{r}_j$ the jth row of the matrix A and by p_j the jth coordinate of the vector $\mathbf{p}$, then the system $A\mathbf{x} = \mathbf{p}$ is the same as having $\mathbf{r}_j \bullet \mathbf{x} = p_j$ for every value of j. Kaczmarz's method works by producing a sequence of vectors each of which satisfies one of the individual equations $\mathbf{r}_j \bullet \mathbf{x} = p_j$. The first research article to explore the application of algebraic reconstruction techniques to medical imaging was [22], which appeared in 1970. The principal technique employed therein for the reconstruction of images turned out to be the same as Kaczmarz's method. A further elaboration of this approach can be found in [25].

9.2.1 Affine spaces

Before looking at Kaczmarz's method itself, we make the following definition.

Definition 9.1. For a fixed n-dimensional vector $\mathbf{r}$ and a number p, the *affine space* $\mathcal{S}_{\mathbf{r},p}$ is defined by

$$\mathcal{S}_{\mathbf{r},p} = \{\mathbf{x} \in \mathbb{R}^n : \mathbf{r} \bullet \mathbf{x} = p\} \ .$$

Note that the affine space $\mathcal{S}_{\mathbf{r},p}$ is a subspace of $\mathbb{R}^n$ if, and only if, $p = 0$.

We have already seen an important example of affine spaces in the lines $\ell_{t,\theta}$. Each point on $\ell_{t,\theta}$ is the terminal point of a vector $\mathbf{x} = \langle t\cos(\theta) - s\sin(\theta), t\sin(\theta) + s\cos(\theta) \rangle$ for some value of the parameter s. Letting $\mathbf{r} = \langle \cos(\theta), \sin(\theta) \rangle$, we compute

$$\begin{aligned} \mathbf{r} \bullet \mathbf{x} &= t\cos^2(\theta) - s\sin(\theta)\cos(\theta) + t\sin^2(\theta) + s\cos(\theta)\sin(\theta) \\ &= t(\cos^2(\theta) + \sin^2(\theta)) \\ &= t \end{aligned}$$

regardless of the value of s. Thus, each line $\ell_{t,\theta}$ is an affine space. If $t = 0$, then $\ell_{0,\theta}$ is a line through the origin and, so, is a subspace of $\mathbb{R}^2$.

Every affine space can be viewed as a copy of a subspace that has been shifted by a fixed vector. For example, for each fixed value of θ, the line

$$\ell_{0,\theta} = \{ \langle -s\sin(\theta), s\cos(\theta) \rangle : -\infty < s < \infty \}$$

forms a subspace of $\mathbb{R}^2$. For each real number t, we then have that

$$\ell_{t,\theta} = \langle t\cos(\theta), t\sin(\theta) \rangle + \ell_{0,\theta} \ .$$

To formulate the same notion slightly differently, let $\mathbf{r} = \langle \cos(\theta), \sin(\theta) \rangle$ and $\mathbf{x}_0 = \langle t\cos(\theta), t\sin(\theta) \rangle$. Then $\mathbf{r} \bullet \mathbf{x}_0 = t$. The subspace $\ell_{0,\theta}$ consists of the set of all vectors $\mathbf{x}$ for which $\mathbf{r} \bullet \mathbf{x} = 0$. Thus, the line $\ell_{t,\theta}$ consists of the terminal points of all vectors of the form $\mathbf{x}_0 + \mathbf{x}$, where $\mathbf{r} \bullet \mathbf{x} = 0$.

Similarly, for any vector $\mathbf{r}$ and any real number p, consider the affine space $\mathcal{S}_{\mathbf{r},p}$ and the subspace $\mathcal{S}_{\mathbf{r},0}$. Observe that, for $\mathbf{x}_0$ and $\mathbf{x}_1$ in $\mathcal{S}_{\mathbf{r},p}$, the vector $\mathbf{x}_h = \mathbf{x}_1 - \mathbf{x}_0$ satisfies the homogeneous equation $\mathbf{r} \bullet \mathbf{x}_h = 0$. That is, $\mathbf{x}_h$ is in the subspace $\mathcal{S}_{\mathbf{r},0}$. Since $\mathbf{x}_1 = \mathbf{x}_h + \mathbf{x}_0$, it follows that every element of the affine space $\mathcal{S}_{\mathbf{r},p}$ can be obtained by adding the vector $\mathbf{x}_0$ to some element of the subspace $\mathcal{S}_{\mathbf{r},0}$. This is reminiscent of the use of a particular solution together with the general homogeneous solution to obtain the general solution to a nonhomogeneous linear differential equation or a nonhomogeneous system of linear equations.

A final crucial observation is that, since the vector $\mathbf{r}$ is orthogonal to the subspace $\mathcal{S}_{\mathbf{r},0}$, and, since the affine space $\mathcal{S}_{\mathbf{r},p}$ is a parallel translation of this subspace, then it follows that the vector $\mathbf{r}$ itself is orthogonal to the affine space $\mathcal{S}_{\mathbf{r},p}$.

Definition 9.2. Affine projection. Given a vector $\mathbf{u}$ and an affine space $\mathcal{S}_{\mathbf{r},p}$ for some vector $\mathbf{r}$ and some number p, the *affine projection* of $\mathbf{u}$ in $\mathcal{S}_{\mathbf{r},p}$ is the vector $\mathbf{u}_*$ in $\mathcal{S}_{\mathbf{r},p}$ that is *closest* to $\mathbf{u}$ amongst all vectors in $\mathcal{S}_{\mathbf{r},p}$.

Now, in order to move from $\mathbf{u}$ to the closest point in the affine space, it is evident that we should move *orthogonally* to the affine space. According to our previous observations, this means that we should move in the direction of the vector $\mathbf{r}$ itself. Thus, the vector $\mathbf{u}_*$ that we seek should have the form $\mathbf{u}_* = \mathbf{u} - \lambda \mathbf{r}$ for some number λ.

Substituting $\mathbf{u}_* = \mathbf{u} - \lambda \mathbf{r}$ into the equation $\mathbf{r} \bullet \mathbf{u}_* = p$ and solving for λ yields

$$\lambda = \frac{(\mathbf{r} \bullet \mathbf{u}) - p}{\mathbf{r} \bullet \mathbf{r}}.$$

Thus, we have proven the following proposition.

Proposition 9.3. *The affine projection $\mathbf{u}_*$ of the vector $\mathbf{u}$ in the affine space $\mathcal{S}_{\mathbf{r},p}$ is given by*

$$\mathbf{u}_* = \mathbf{u} - \left(\frac{(\mathbf{r} \bullet \mathbf{u}) - p}{\mathbf{r} \bullet \mathbf{r}} \right) \mathbf{r}. \tag{9.7}$$

9.2.2 Kaczmarz's method

Now we put our knowledge of affine spaces to work. In matrix form, let A denote the $J \times K^2$ matrix whose ith row is given by the vector $\mathbf{r}_i$, and take $\mathbf{p}$ to be the column vector with ith coordinate p_i, for $i = 1, \ldots, J$. Then the equation $A\mathbf{x} = \mathbf{p}$ describes the linear system in (9.6). Recall that our goal is to find an approximate solution to a linear system $A\mathbf{x} = \mathbf{p}$. Again denote the ith row of A by $\mathbf{r}_i$ and the ith coordinate of $\mathbf{p}$ by p_i. Then each of the equations $\mathbf{r}_i \bullet \mathbf{x} = p_i$ describes an affine space. Kaczmarz's method proceeds by starting with an initial guess at a solution, a vector of prospective color values, and then computing the affine projection of this initial guess onto the first affine space in our list. This projection is then projected onto the next affine space in the list, and so on until we have gone through the entire list of affine spaces. This constitutes one iteration. The result of this iteration becomes the starting point for the next iteration.

In detail, the method proceeds as follows.

(i)   Select a starting guess for $\mathbf{x}$; call it $\mathbf{x}^0$.

(ii) Next set $\mathbf{x}^{0,0} = \mathbf{x}^0$.

(iii)   The inductive step is this: Once the vector $\mathbf{x}^{0,j-1}$ has been determined, define

$$\mathbf{x}^{0,j} = \mathbf{x}^{0,j-1} - \left(\frac{\mathbf{x}^{0,j-1} \bullet \mathbf{r}_j - p_j}{\mathbf{r}_j \bullet \mathbf{r}_j} \right) \mathbf{r}_j . \tag{9.8}$$

We have used the affine projection formula (9.7) from Proposition 9.3.

(iv)   Note that if the matrix A has J rows, then the vectors $\mathbf{x}^{0,1}$, $\mathbf{x}^{0,2}$, ..., $\mathbf{x}^{0,J}$ will be computed.

(v)   Once $\mathbf{x}^{0,J}$ has been computed, define $\mathbf{x}^1 = \mathbf{x}^{0,J}$ and begin the process again starting with $\mathbf{x}^1$. That is, now set $\mathbf{x}^{1,0} = \mathbf{x}^1$ and compute the vectors $\mathbf{x}^{1,1}$, $\mathbf{x}^{1,2}$, ..., $\mathbf{x}^{1,J}$, as in (9.8).

(vi)   Then let $\mathbf{x}^2 = \mathbf{x}^{1,J}$ and repeat the process starting with $\mathbf{x}^{2,0} = \mathbf{x}^2$.

(vii)   Stop when we've had enough!

There are, as we might expect, some computational concerns with this method. In principle, the successive vectors $\mathbf{x}^0$, $\mathbf{x}^1$, $\mathbf{x}^2$, ... should get closer to a vector that satisfies the original system $A\mathbf{x} = \mathbf{p}$. However, the convergence may be quite slow, meaning that many steps of the iteration would have to be applied to get a good approximant. Also, if the system has no solution, then the vectors computed from the algorithm might settle into a specific pattern, called an attractor in dynamical systems theory, or might even exhibit chaotic behavior.

Example 9.4. Apply Kaczmarz's method to the system consisting of just the two lines $x + 2y = 5$ and $x - y = 1$. So $\mathbf{r}_1 = \langle 1, 2 \rangle$, $\mathbf{r}_2 = \langle 1, -1 \rangle$, $p_1 = 5$, and $p_2 = 1$. With the initial guess $\mathbf{x}^0 = \langle 0.5, 0.5 \rangle$, the diagram on the left in Figure 9.1 shows that the solution $\langle 7/3, 4/3 \rangle$ will quickly be found.

However, when we include the third line $4x + y = 6$ (so $\mathbf{r}_3 = \langle 4, 1 \rangle$ and $p_3 = 6$), then the successive iterations settle into a triangular pattern, shown in the diagram on the right in the figure.

Example with R 9.5. In an implementation of Kaczmarz's method, one can choose to save only the last estimate of the solution, after all cycles have been completed. Alternatively, one can generate a matrix where each successive row is an intermediate estimate, either from a single equation or from a full cycle. We present two versions here. The first approach is applied to the systems of equations in Example 9.4 and was used to produce Figure 9.1.

```
##Kaczmarz method: save next estimate from each eqn.
kacz.v0=function(mat,rhs,ncycles){
neq=nrow(mat)
V=matrix(double((neq*ncycles+1)*ncol(mat)),
neq*ncycles+1,ncol(mat))
V[1,]=rep(0.5,2)
for (i in 1:ncycles){
for (j in 1:neq){
```

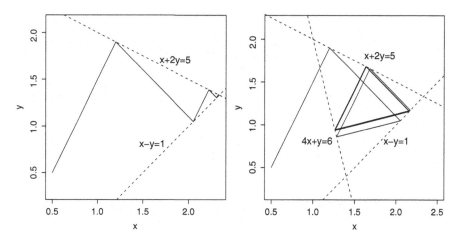

Fig. 9.1. On the left, Kaczmarz's method converges quickly to the point of intersection of two lines. On the right, the successive iterations settle into a triangular pattern for a system of three lines.

```
V[neq*(i-1)+j+1,]=ifelse(mat[j,]==0,V[neq*(i-1)+j,],
V[neq*(i-1)+j,]-((sum(V[neq*(i-1)+j,]*mat[j,])-
rhs[j])/sum(mat[j,]*mat[j,]))*mat[j,])}}
list(V=V)}
##For Figure 09_1
R1=matrix(c(1,2,1,-1),2,2,byrow=T)#2 lines
p1=c(5,1)
V1=kacz.v0(R1,p1,2)$V
R2=matrix(c(1,2,1,-1,4,1),3,2,byrow=T)#3 lines
p2=c(5,1,6)
V2=kacz.v0(R2,p2,3)$V
#plot fig09_1a
plot(V1[,1],V1[,2],type="l",lwd=2,xlab="x",ylab="y")
plot(V2[,1],V2[,2],type="l",asp=1,xlab="x",ylab="y",lwd=2)
```

In our second version of Kaczmarz's method, all intermediate estimates are computed, but only the final estimate is saved. This version will be used in the CT scan image reconstructions that follow.

```
##Kaczmarz's method; save only most recent estimate
kaczmarz.basic=function(mat,rhs,numcycles){
numeq=nrow(mat)
sol.est=rep(0.5,ncol(mat))#initial "guess" of all 0.5s
for (i in 1:numcycles){
for (j in 1:numeq){
sol.est=ifelse(mat[j,]==0,sol.est,sol.est-
((sum(sol.est*mat[j,])-rhs[j])/sum(mat[j,]*mat[j,]))*
   mat[j,])
}}list(sol.est=sol.est)}
```

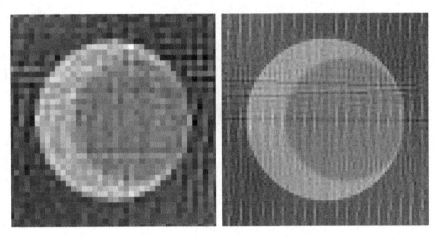

Fig. 9.2. Kaczmarz's method applied to a crescent-shaped phantom: On the left, a 40×40 image grid and 2460 values of the Radon transform; on the right, a 100×100 image grid and 9090 values of the Radon transform.

Before looking at an image created using Kaczmarz's method, we state, without proof, the main convergence theorem for this algorithm. (For a proof, see [17] or [39].)

Theorem 9.6. *If the linear system* $A\mathbf{x} = \mathbf{p}$ *has at least one solution, then Kaczmarz's method converges to a solution of this system. Moreover, if* $\mathbf{x}^0$ *is in the range of* A^T *, then Kaczmarz's method converges to the solution of minimum norm.*

The convergence result in Theorem 9.6 generally is not relevant in medical imaging, where the linear systems encountered tend to be indeterminate and where, in any case, it is computationally feasible to run only a few iterations of Kazcmarz's method.

The images in Figure 9.2 are reconstructions of the crescent-shaped phantom illustrated in Figure 2.8 and defined by the attenuation function in (2.11). For each image, five full iterations of Kaczmarz's method were applied with an initial vector $\mathbf{x}^0$ having every coordinate equal to 0.5. (In other words, the starting point was taken to be a neutral grey image.) For the coarser image, the Radon transform of the phantom was sampled using $\Delta t = 0.05$ on the interval $-1 \le t \le 1$, with angle increments of $\Delta \theta = \pi/60$, for a total of 2460 different values. The corresponding system of equations, (9.6), is overdetermined in this case. The second image has a grid with 10000 pixels and used $\Delta t = .02$ and $\Delta \theta = \pi/90$, for a total of 9090 values of the Radon transform. With these settings, the system (9.6) is underdetermined. These images show the crescent, but do not necessarily compare favorably to the reconstructions in Figures 8.8 and 8.9.

Example with R 9.7. To create an image from X-ray data using Kaczmarz's method, as in Figure 9.2, we must compute the matrix whose entries are the lengths of the intersections of the lines in the scan with the pixels in the image grid. Since each pixel is a small square, we can follow the basic approach from Example 2.15 above to compute each entry of the coefficient matrix. In R, it is convenient to encode this as a function of the set of lines and the locations of the pixels. For instance, if the general procedure is `radon.pix`, then the output for a specific scan and selected image grid might be

```
rad.mat=radon.pix(grid.theta,grid.t,grid.cx,grid.cy)$coef.
```

Next, the right-hand sides are the X-ray data values from the scan, or, in this exercise, the values of the Radon transform of a phantom. Notice that the coefficient matrix can be re-used, while the right-hand sides will change with each scan. The color values for the image are computed by applying the procedure `kaczmarz.basic` from Example 9.5. (In this exercise, `rad.mat` is the coefficient matrix just computed and `rp1` is the vector of X-ray data for the phantom. Then `image.mat` is the matrix of color values.)

```
sys2=kaczmarz.basic(rad.mat,rp1,5)$sol.est
image.mat=matrix((sys2-min(sys2))/(max(sys2)-min(sys2)),
nrow=K,byrow=T)
```

Finally, we plot each pixel using the `polygon` command, seen in Example 1.1. This time, each square pixel is its own polygon. The grid is defined by the sets `xval` and `yval` of x- and y-coordinates, respectively.

```
plot(c(-1,1), c(-1,1), type = "n",axes="",asp=1)
for (i in 1:K){
for (j in 1:K){
polygon(c(xval[j],xval[j+1],xval[j+1],xval[j],xval[j]),
c(yval[i],yval[i],yval[i+1],yval[i+1],i),
col = gray(image.mat[i,j]),border = NA)}}
```

One concern about the use of Kaczmarz's method in the context of tomography, as mentioned before, is that the sheer size of the system of equations involved can be an impediment. Also, each of the values r_{jk} represents the length of the intersection of one of the X-ray beams with one of the pixel squares in the image grid. Thus, as observed before, most of these values are zeros. The formula for computing $\mathbf{x}^{k,j}$ from $\mathbf{x}^{k,j-1}$ only alters $\mathbf{x}^{k,j-1}$ in those components that correspond to the pixels through which the jth beam passes. To streamline the computation of $\mathbf{x}^{k,j-1} \bullet \mathbf{r}_j$, we could store the locations of the nonzero entries of $\mathbf{r}_j$. In its favor, Kaczmarz's method can be applied to the fan beam and cone beam geometries without re-binning the scanner data, since each X-ray in the scan simply defines another affine subspace in the system.

9.2.3 Variations of Kaczmarz's method

Perhaps the most commonly employed variation of Kaczmarz's method involves the introduction of so-called *relaxation parameters* in the crucial step (9.8) of the algorithm. Specifically, for each j and k, let λ_{jk} satisfy $0 < \lambda_{jk} < 2$ and replace the formula in (9.8) with the formula

$$\mathbf{x}^{k,j} = \mathbf{x}^{k,j-1} - \lambda_{jk} \cdot \left(\frac{\mathbf{x}^{k,j-1} \bullet \mathbf{r}_j - p_j}{\mathbf{r}_j \bullet \mathbf{r}_j} \right) \mathbf{r}_j. \tag{9.9}$$

For $\lambda_{jk} = 1$ this is the same as before. For $0 < \lambda_{jk} < 1$, the vector $\mathbf{x}^{k,j-1}$ is projected only part of the way to the affine space $\mathcal{S}_{\mathbf{r}_j, p_j}$. When $1 < \lambda_{jk} < 2$, the vector $\mathbf{x}^{k,j-1}$ is projected to the other side of $\mathcal{S}_{\mathbf{r}_j, p_j}$. Note that, if $\lambda_{jk} = 2$, then the vector $\mathbf{x}^{k,j}$ is just the reflection of $\mathbf{x}^{k,j-1}$ across $\mathcal{S}_{\mathbf{r}_j, p_j}$ and there is no improvement in the proximity to a solution. This is the reason for the restriction $\lambda_{jk} < 2$. In fact, the usual requirement is that the value of λ_{jk} be bounded away from 0 and 2; that is, there should be numbers α and β such that $0 < \alpha \leq \lambda_{jk} \leq \beta < 2$ for all j and k. The picture on the left in Figure 9.3 shows a reconstruction of a phantom using Kaczmarz's method, where the relaxation parameter at each step is a number between 0.5 and 1.5 that was chosen randomly from a uniform distribution. The result is virtually indistinguishable from the reconstruction using the basic Kaczmarz method, shown on the right in Figure 9.2.

Example with R 9.8. Relaxation parameters can be introduced into the computer implementation of Kaczmarz's method with a simple modifcation to the procedure in 9.5. For instance, the relaxation parameter can be chosen randomly at each step, like so.

```
#Kaczmarz's method with relaxation
kaczmarz.relax=function(mat,rhs,numcycles){
numeq=nrow(mat)
solB=rep(0.5,ncol(mat))
for (j in 1:numcycles){
for (i in 1:numeq){
solB=ifelse(mat[i,]==0,solB,solB-runif(1,min=0.5,max=1.5)*
((sum(solB*mat[i,])-rhs[i])/sum(mat[i,]*mat[i,]))*mat[i,])}}
list(solB=solB)}
```

Then continue as before to compute the coefficient matrix and so on.

The additional control over the projection offered by the relaxation parameters can be used to facilitate finding an acceptable approximate solution to an indeterminate system. Alternatively, we can use this additional control to modify the original system of linear equations by replacing it with a system of inequalities instead. To do this, we select, for each j, a (small) positive number ε_j and consider the inequalities

$$p_j - \varepsilon_j \leq \mathbf{r}_j \bullet \mathbf{x} \leq p_j + \varepsilon_j .$$

A solution to this system of inequalities is a vector $\mathbf{x}^*$ that, instead of lying in the intersection of some collection of affine spaces, lies in close proximity to those spaces. Geometrically, if we think of an affine space as a higher-dimensional plane sitting inside a many-dimensional space, then vectors in proximity to an affine space form a higher-dimensional slab, with thickness $2 \cdot \varepsilon_j$. The solution vector $\mathbf{x}^*$ would lie inside these slabs. The use of relaxation parameters in the variation of Kaczmarz's method enables us to control the projection of each successive vector in the iteration into the next slab. When inequalities are used instead of equations, the problem is called a *feasibility problem* rather than an optimization problem. For the picture on the right in Figure 9.3, random noise, from a Gaussian with mean 0 and standard deviation 0.02, was added to each value of the Radon transform (the p_j in the application of Kaczmarz's method).

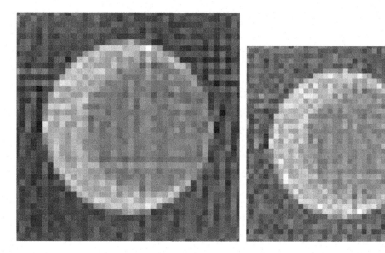

Fig. 9.3. Variations of Kaczmarz's method: On the left, the relaxation parameter at each step is a number between 0.5 and 1.5 chosen randomly from a uniform distribution; on the right, random Gaussian noise has been added to the values of the Radon transform.

The article [11] provides a nice introduction to these ideas, while [10] and [22] offer more details of these methods. A much more general approach to feasibility problems that includes Kaczmarz's method and its variants can be found in the comprehensive article [3].

9.3   Least squares approximation

For a given $M \times N$ matrix A and a given vector $\mathbf{p}$ in $\mathbb{R}^M$, the system $A\mathbf{x} = \mathbf{p}$ may not have a solution. One approach to finding an approximate solution is to find the vector $\widehat{\mathbf{y}}$ of the form $\widehat{\mathbf{y}} = A\widehat{\mathbf{x}}$ such that $\widehat{\mathbf{y}}$ is *closest* to $\mathbf{p}$ amongst all vectors of this form. Thus, the goal of least squares approximation is to find a vector $\widehat{\mathbf{x}}$ in $\mathbb{R}^N$ such that

$$||A\widehat{\mathbf{x}} - \mathbf{p}|| = \min_{\mathbf{x} \in \mathbb{R}^N} ||A\mathbf{x} - \mathbf{p}||. \tag{9.10}$$

In other words, we wish to find the vector $A\widehat{\mathbf{x}}$ in the range of the matrix A that is closest to $\mathbf{p}$ amongst all elements of the range of A. Because the magnitude of a vector can be expressed as a sum of squares, this form of approximation is called *least squares approximation*.

Geometrically, if we take an arbitrary element $A\mathbf{x}$ in the range of A and consider the projection of the vector $(A\mathbf{x} - \mathbf{p})$ onto the range of A, then the foot of this projection will be a vector in the range of A that is at least as close to $\mathbf{p}$ as the original vector $A\mathbf{x}$ was. Thus, the closest element to $\mathbf{p}$ in the range of A is the element $A\widehat{\mathbf{x}}$ for which the foot of the projection of $(A\widehat{\mathbf{x}} - \mathbf{p})$ onto the range of A is the vector $A\widehat{\mathbf{x}}$ itself. This means that the vector $(A\widehat{\mathbf{x}} - \mathbf{p})$ must be orthogonal to the range of A. By Corollary B.8 in Appendix B, this means that the vector $(A\widehat{\mathbf{x}} - \mathbf{p})$ must lie in the nullspace of the matrix A^T. In other words, the vector $\widehat{\mathbf{x}}$ must satisfy the equation

$$A^T \left(A\widehat{\mathbf{x}} - \mathbf{p} \right) = 0 \,, \tag{9.11}$$

or what is the same thing,

$$A^T A\widehat{\mathbf{x}} = A^T \mathbf{p}. \tag{9.12}$$

This last equation is called the *normal equation*.

Definition 9.9. A *least squares solution* to the equation $A\mathbf{x} = \mathbf{p}$ is a vector $\widehat{\mathbf{x}}$ that satisfies the normal equation (9.12). In this case, the vector $A\widehat{\mathbf{x}}$ is the closest element in the range of A to the vector $\mathbf{p}$.

Notice that, in the case where the matrix $A^T A$ is invertible, then the normal equation (9.12) yields the least squares solution

$$\widehat{\mathbf{x}} = \left(A^T A \right)^{-1} A^T \mathbf{p}. \tag{9.13}$$

In general, however, $A^T A$ need not be invertible, in which case the least squares solution $\widehat{\mathbf{x}}$ is not unique. Nonetheless, the range element $\widehat{\mathbf{y}} = A\widehat{\mathbf{x}}$ that is closest to $\mathbf{p}$ is unique.

Example 9.10. Take $A = \begin{bmatrix} -1 & 2 \\ 2 & -3 \\ -1 & 3 \end{bmatrix}$ and $\mathbf{p} = \begin{bmatrix} 4 \\ 1 \\ 2 \end{bmatrix}$. Show that $A^T A$ is invertible and that

the (unique) least squares solution, computed from (9.13), is $\widehat{\mathbf{x}} = \begin{bmatrix} 3 \\ 2 \end{bmatrix}$. Compute $||A\widehat{\mathbf{x}} - \mathbf{p}||$

in this case.

Example 9.11. Take $A = \begin{bmatrix} 1 & 1 & 0 \\ 1 & 1 & 0 \\ 1 & 0 & 1 \\ 1 & 0 & 1 \end{bmatrix}$ and $\mathbf{p} = \begin{bmatrix} 1 \\ 3 \\ 8 \\ 2 \end{bmatrix}$. Show that $A^T A$ is not invertible. Find

all solutions to the normal equation (9.12) and show that the (unique) element closest to $\mathbf{p}$

in the range of A is $\widehat{\mathbf{y}} = \begin{bmatrix} 2 \\ 2 \\ 5 \\ 5 \end{bmatrix}$. Compute $||\widehat{\mathbf{y}} - \mathbf{p}||$ in this case.

Here is an alternate approach to solving the least squares approximation problem that leads us again to the normal equation (9.12). For a given $M \times N$ matrix A and a given vector $\mathbf{p}$ in $\mathbb{R}^M$, define a real-number-valued function $F : \mathbb{R}^N \to \mathbb{R}$ by

$$F(\mathbf{x}) := ||A\mathbf{x} - \mathbf{p}||^2 = (A\mathbf{x} - \mathbf{p}) \bullet (A\mathbf{x} - \mathbf{p}) \,, \text{ for all } \mathbf{x} \text{ in } \mathbb{R}^N .$$

One can show that the *gradient vector* of F satisfies

$$\nabla F(\mathbf{x}) = 2 \left(A^T A \mathbf{x} - A^T \mathbf{p} \right) , \text{ for all } \mathbf{x} \text{ in } \mathbb{R}^N . \tag{9.14}$$

The least squares solution $\widehat{\mathbf{x}}$ produces a minimum value for F and, hence, the gradient of F at $\widehat{\mathbf{x}}$ must vanish. That is, $\nabla F(\widehat{\mathbf{x}}) = \mathbf{0}$ for the least squares solution $\widehat{\mathbf{x}}$. According to (9.14), then, the least squares solution $\widehat{\mathbf{x}}$ satisfies the normal equation $A^T A \widehat{\mathbf{x}} = A^T \mathbf{p}$.

One computational concern associated with the least squares method in the context of imaging is that the matrix $A^T A$ in the normal equation (9.12) is huge, on the order of K^2-by-K^2. Also, the matrix $A^T A$ might not be sparse even though A is. Another concern is that the matrix $A^T A$ might not be invertible or that its inverse might be difficult to compute. Moreover, round-off errors can be fatal. For instance, a matrix entry that ought to be 0 but shows up as a tiny nonzero number can wreck the process of inverting a matrix. Similarly, an entry that ought to be a tiny nonzero number but shows up as 0 can also have a deleterious effect.

9.4 Pseudoinverses and least squares

Returning to the problem of minimizing $||A\mathbf{x}-\mathbf{p}||$, suppose $\mathbf{x}_0$ and $\mathbf{x}_1$ are any two solutions to the normal equation, $A^T A \mathbf{x} = A^T \mathbf{p}$. Then $A^T A(\mathbf{x}_0 - \mathbf{x}_1) = \mathbf{0}$. That is, the difference $(\mathbf{x}_0 - \mathbf{x}_1)$ lies in the nullspace of $A^T A$. From Theorem B.9, this means that $(\mathbf{x}_0 - \mathbf{x}_1)$ is in the nullspace of A. It follows that there is a *unique* solution to the normal equation that is also orthogonal to the nullspace of A. (If there were two such solutions, then their difference would be in the nullspace of A and at the same time orthogonal to the nullspace of A; so their difference would have to be $\mathbf{0}$.) Let's denote this special solution by $\mathbf{x}^+$. Importantly, *the norm of $\mathbf{x}^+$ is as small as possible for solutions of the normal equation.* This is so because, as we just saw, any other solution must differ from $\mathbf{x}^+$ by a component in the nullspace of A, orthogonal to $\mathbf{x}^+$. Adding this orthogonal component can only increase the norm, by the Pythagorean theorem. This uniquely determined vector $\mathbf{x}^+$ is called the *Moore–Penrose* solution to the normal equation. Note that $\mathbf{x}^+$ lies in the range of A^T, from Corollary B.8.

When the matrix $A^T A$ happens to be invertible, then the nullspace of $A^T A$, and, so, too, the nullspace of A, consists just of the zero vector. In this case, as we observed earlier, the normal equation (9.12) yields the unique least squares solution $\mathbf{x}^+ = \left(A^T A \right)^{-1} A^T \mathbf{p}$, which coincides with the Moore–Penrose solution.

Example 9.12. Going back to Example 9.11, let $A = \begin{bmatrix} 1 & 1 & 0 \\ 1 & 1 & 0 \\ 1 & 0 & 1 \\ 1 & 0 & 1 \end{bmatrix}$ and $\mathbf{p} = (1, 3, 8, 2)$. In

this case, $A^T A$ is not invertible. The nullspace of A is the set $\{t(-1, 1, 1) : t \in \mathbb{R}\}$ and the set of solutions to the corresponding normal equation is given by $\{(5, -3, 0) + t(-1, 1, 1) :$

$t \in \mathbb{R}$}. The norm of a typical solution is $\sqrt{(5-t)^2 + (-3+t)^2 + t^2}$, which is minimized when $t = 8/3$. Thus, the Moore–Penrose solution is $\mathbf{x}^+ = (5, -3, 0) + (8/3)(-1, 1, 1) = (7/3, -1/3, 8/3)$. Note that this is, indeed, orthogonal to the vector $(-1, 1, 1)$ and, hence, to the nullspace of A.

To find the Moore–Penrose solution $\mathbf{x}^+$ in Example 9.12, we first found the general solution to the normal equation $A^T A \mathbf{x} = A^T \mathbf{p}$ and then figured out which solution had the minimum possible norm. A different approach is based on the singular value decomposition, discussed in Appendix B. (See (B.5), (B.6), and (B.7).)

Using the singular value decomposition (SVD) of A, we can rewrite our original equation, $A\mathbf{x} = \mathbf{p}$, as $U\Sigma V^T \mathbf{x} = \mathbf{p}$. Pretending for a moment that the matrix Σ is invertible (though we have no right to think this would be so!), we get the "solution" $\mathbf{x} = V"\Sigma^{-1}"U^T\mathbf{p}$, where "$\Sigma^{-1}$" is in quotation marks to remind us that it is possibly fictitious. But what *would* "Σ^{-1}" look like if it *did* exist? Well, where Σ has the entry σ_j on its diagonal, now we would want the reciprocal value $1/\sigma_j$. This is impossible, of course, when $\sigma_j = 0$. Nonetheless, let's push this idea as far as it can go: Given our $M \times N$ matrix Σ, let Σ^+ denote the $N \times M$ matrix with diagonal entry $1/\sigma_j$ whenever $\sigma_j \neq 0$ and 0 whenever $\sigma_j = 0$. (That is, we just leave any 0s on the diagonal of Σ as they are, take reciprocals of the nonzero entries, and transpose the whole thing.) This matrix Σ^+ is called the *pseudoinverse* of Σ. Each of the matrix products $\Sigma^+\Sigma$ and $\Sigma\Sigma^+$ has an $r \times r$ identity matrix in its upper left corner, where r is the number of nonzero singular values. Now define the *pseudoinverse* of the matrix A by

$$A^+ = V\Sigma^+ U^T.$$

The Moore–Penrose solution to the normal equation is now given by

$$\mathbf{x}^+ = A^+\mathbf{p} = \left(V\Sigma^+ U^T\right)\mathbf{p}.$$

To see that this really works, we compute

$$\begin{aligned}
A^T A\mathbf{x}^+ &= \left(A^T A V\right) \Sigma^+ U^T\mathbf{p} \\
&= VD\Sigma^+ U^T\mathbf{p} \text{ (since } A^T A = VDV^{-1}) \\
&= V\Sigma^T U^T\mathbf{p} \text{ (since } D\Sigma^+ = \Sigma^T) \\
&= A^T\mathbf{p} \text{ (since } A^T = \left(U\Sigma V^T\right)^T = V\Sigma^T U^T).
\end{aligned}$$

Thus, $\mathbf{x}^+$ satisfies the normal equation. Moreover, $\mathbf{x}^+$ is, by its definition, a linear combination of those columns of V that correspond to the *nonzero* singular values of A. The subspace spanned by these columns of V is orthogonal to the nullspace of A, which is spanned by the remaining columns of V. Therefore, the vector $\mathbf{x}^+$ is orthogonal to the nullspace of A, which is the other property required of the Moore–Penrose solution to the normal equation.

Example 9.13. Returning to Example 9.12, we take $A = \begin{bmatrix} 1 & 1 & 0 \\ 1 & 1 & 0 \\ 1 & 0 & 1 \\ 1 & 0 & 1 \end{bmatrix}$ and $\mathbf{p} = (1, 3, 8, 2)$,

and we consider the equation $A\mathbf{x} = \mathbf{p}$. Example B.11, in Appendix B, shows that $A^T A$ has the eigenvalue decomposition $A^T A = VDV^T$, where

$$D = \begin{bmatrix} 6 & 0 & 0 \\ 0 & 2 & 0 \\ 0 & 0 & 0 \end{bmatrix} \text{ and } V = \begin{bmatrix} 2/\sqrt{6} & 0 & -1/\sqrt{3} \\ 1/\sqrt{6} & -1/\sqrt{2} & 1/\sqrt{3} \\ 1/\sqrt{6} & 1/\sqrt{2} & 1/\sqrt{3} \end{bmatrix}.$$

Next we compute two units vectors, $\mathbf{u}_1$ and $\mathbf{u}_2$, such that $A\mathbf{v}_1 = \sqrt{6}\mathbf{u}_1$ and $A\mathbf{v}_2 = \sqrt{2}\mathbf{u}_2$. Two additional unit vectors, $\mathbf{u}_3$ and $\mathbf{u}_4$ are chosen to produce a full orthonormal basis for $\mathbb{R}^4$. This yields the matrix

$$U = \begin{bmatrix} 1/2 & -1/2 & 1/\sqrt{2} & 0 \\ 1/2 & -1/2 & -1/\sqrt{2} & 0 \\ 1/2 & 1/2 & 0 & 1/\sqrt{2} \\ 1/2 & 1/2 & 0 & -1/\sqrt{2} \end{bmatrix}$$

as one possibility. With

$$\Sigma = \begin{bmatrix} \sqrt{6} & 0 & 0 \\ 0 & \sqrt{2} & 0 \\ 0 & 0 & 0 \\ 0 & 0 & 0 \end{bmatrix},$$

the singular value decomposition of A is now given by $U\Sigma V^T$. The two pseudoinverses are

$$\Sigma^+ = \begin{bmatrix} 1/\sqrt{6} & 0 & 0 & 0 \\ 0 & 1/\sqrt{2} & 0 & 0 \\ 0 & 0 & 0 & 0 \end{bmatrix},$$

and $A^+ = V\Sigma^+ U^T = \begin{bmatrix} 1/6 & 1/6 & 1/6 & 1/6 \\ 1/3 & 1/3 & -1/6 & -1/6 \\ -1/6 & -1/6 & 1/3 & 1/3 \end{bmatrix}.$

Finally, we compute the Moore–Penrose solution as

$$\mathbf{x}^+ = A^+\mathbf{p} = \begin{bmatrix} 1/6 & 1/6 & 1/6 & 1/6 \\ 1/3 & 1/3 & -1/6 & -1/6 \\ -1/6 & -1/6 & 1/3 & 1/3 \end{bmatrix} \begin{bmatrix} 1 \\ 3 \\ 8 \\ 2 \end{bmatrix} = \begin{bmatrix} 7/3 \\ -1/3 \\ 8/3 \end{bmatrix}.$$

Happily, this agrees with our earlier solution!

Example with R 9.14. The singular value decomposition of a matrix is available in R with the `svd()` command. This returns the three factors, which can be called separately. The pseudoinverse is also available by loading the MASS package and using the command `ginv()`. The preceding example is computed as follows.

```
##SVD; pseudoinverse of a matrix
A=matrix(c(1,1,1,1,1,1,0,0,0,0,1,1),nrow=4)
p=matrix(c(1,3,8,2))
A0=svd(A)#yields 3 factors u, d, v
A1=round(A0$u%*%diag(A0$d)%*%t(A0$v),5)
#load package MASS; #then ginv() is pseudoinverse
Aplus=ginv(A)
xplus=Aplus%*%p#Moore--Penrose solution
```

For a problem as small as the one in Examples 9.12 and 9.13, all of this machinery may seem overwhelming. Isn't it hard to find the eigenvalues of a matrix that's larger than 2×2? So isn't the singular value decomposition hard to compute? It didn't seem that bad to just solve the normal equation using our familiar, trusted method of Gaussian elimination. These are reasonable concerns. We must keep in mind that the systems of equations we typically encounter in CT imaging are large, with sparse coefficient matrices. Solving the normal equation using Gaussian elimination could get unwieldy, and finding the solution of minimum norm may be an onerous task. So there are potential difficulties with both the Gaussian elimination and the pseudoinverse approaches. To address this, we will look at two popular methods of *approximating* the Moore–Penrose solution that are computationally manageable.

9.5 Spectral filtering and regularization

Truncated SVD A basic approach to simplifying the work of the singular value decomposition is to use just part of it. The geometric point of view discussed in Remark B.12 shows that the largest singular values of A, along with the corresponding columns of V and U, capture the dominant behavior of A. This is particularly relevant if some of the nonzero singular values are quite small relative to the larger ones. For instance, an ellipse with one principal axis of length 100 and the other principal axis of length 1 is not much different than a line segment.

A large disparity in the sizes of the nonzero singular values also distorts the behavior of the pseudoinverse, Σ^+, where the reciprocal of a tiny singular value will tend to dominate the computation of $\mathbf{x}^+$.

Mathematically, we can select the k largest positive singular values and approximate A by $A_k = \sum_{j=1}^{k} \sigma_j \mathbf{u}_j \mathbf{v}_j^T$. Equivalently, $A_k = U_k \Sigma_k V_k^T$, where U_k and V_k are formed from just the first k columns of U and V, respectively, and Σ_k is the $k \times k$ diagonal matrix with diagonal entries $\sigma_1 \geq \ldots \geq \sigma_k > 0$. The $M \times N$ matrix A_k has rank equal to k, where A has rank $r > k$, and is called the *rank k truncated SVD* of A. By retaining the largest singular values of A, the matrix A_k captures much of the behavior of A.

Example 9.15. For the matrix A in Example 9.13, there are only two nonzero singular values, so in this example we'll keep just the largest one, $\sqrt{6}$. This gives us the rank 1 truncated SVD

$$A_1 = \sqrt{6}\mathbf{u}_1\mathbf{v}_1^T = \sqrt{6} \begin{bmatrix} 1/2 \\ 1/2 \\ 1/2 \\ 1/2 \end{bmatrix} \begin{bmatrix} \frac{2}{\sqrt{6}} & \frac{1}{\sqrt{6}} & \frac{1}{\sqrt{6}} \end{bmatrix} = \begin{bmatrix} 1\ 1/2\ 1/2 \\ 1\ 1/2\ 1/2 \\ 1\ 1/2\ 1/2 \\ 1\ 1/2\ 1/2 \end{bmatrix}.$$

The rank 1 matrix A_1 has matrix norm $\|A_1\| = \sqrt{6}$, the same as A, and the difference $(A - A_1)$ has matrix norm $\|A - A_1\| = \sqrt{2}$, equal to the largest singular value not used in the approximation.

We can now also compute a rank 1 approximation to the pseudoinverse as

$$A_1^+ = (1/\sqrt{6})\mathbf{v}_1\mathbf{u}_1^T = \frac{1}{12} \cdot \begin{bmatrix} 2\ 2\ 2\ 2 \\ 1\ 1\ 1\ 1 \\ 1\ 1\ 1\ 1 \end{bmatrix}.$$

With $\mathbf{p} = (1, 3, 8, 2)$ as before, we get $A_1^+\mathbf{p} = (7/3, 7/6, 7/6)$ as our approximation of the Moore–Penrose solution to the normal equation $A^TA\mathbf{x} = A^T\mathbf{p}$. One can debate the quality of this approximation; it seems we may have given up too much by dropping the second-largest singular value, $\sqrt{2}$, which, after all, is not that small relative to $\sqrt{6}$. (The ratio is $\sqrt{6}/\sqrt{2} \approx 1.73$.)

Example 9.16. Perhaps we can get a better sense of the benefits of truncation with an example where there is a greater disparity between the largest and smallest nonzero singular values. (The ratio of these two singular values is called the *condition number* of a matrix; a matrix with a large condition number is a good candidate for using the truncated SVD.) Tweaking Example 9.15, let

$$B = \begin{bmatrix} 1\ 1\ 0\ \ 0.05 \\ 1\ 1\ 0\ -0.05 \\ 1\ 0\ 1\ \ 0.05 \\ 1\ 0\ 1\ -0.05 \end{bmatrix}.$$

The singular value decomposition is $B = U \Sigma V^T$, where

$$\Sigma = \begin{bmatrix} \sqrt{6} & 0 & 0 & 0 \\ 0 & \sqrt{2} & 0 & 0 \\ 0 & 0 & 0.1 & 0 \\ 0 & 0 & 0 & 0 \end{bmatrix}, \quad V = \begin{bmatrix} 2/\sqrt{6} & 0 & 0 & -1/\sqrt{3} \\ 1/\sqrt{6} & -1/\sqrt{2} & 0 & 1/\sqrt{3} \\ 1/\sqrt{6} & 1/\sqrt{2} & 0 & 1/\sqrt{3} \\ 0 & 0 & 1 & 0 \end{bmatrix},$$

$$\text{and } U = \begin{bmatrix} 1/2 & -1/2 & 1/2 & 1/2 \\ 1/2 & -1/2 & -1/2 & -1/2 \\ 1/2 & 1/2 & 1/2 & -1/2 \\ 1/2 & 1/2 & -1/2 & 1/2 \end{bmatrix}.$$

The pseudoinverse is

$$B^+ = \begin{bmatrix} 1/6 & 1/6 & 1/6 & 1/6 \\ 1/3 & 1/3 & -1/6 & -1/6 \\ -1/6 & -1/6 & 1/3 & 1/3 \\ 5 & -5 & 5 & -5 \end{bmatrix}.$$

Once again taking $\mathbf{p} = (1, 3, 8, 2)$, the Moore–Penrose solution to the normal equation $B^T B \mathbf{x} = B^T \mathbf{p}$ is given by $B^+ \mathbf{p} = [7/3 \ {-1/3} \ 8/3 \ 20]^T$. Now let's truncate to get the best rank 2 approximation to B, given by $B_2 = \sqrt{6}\mathbf{u}_1\mathbf{v}_1^T + \sqrt{2}\mathbf{u}_2\mathbf{v}_2^T$. This is the same as B except the fourth column is now all 0s. The pseudoinverse B_2^+, correspondingly, is the same as B^+ except that the bottom row is now all 0s. Thus, we can approximate the Moore–Penrose solution as $\mathbf{x}_2^+ = B_2^+ \mathbf{p} = [7/3 \ {-1/3} \ 8/3 \ 0]^T$. Comparing $B^T B\mathbf{x}_2^+$ to $B^T\mathbf{p}$, we find that the difference is the vector $[0 \ \ 0 \ \ 0 \ \ 1/5]^T$, which has length $1/5$; so this approximation is pretty good. Tossing out the smallest nonzero singular value didn't cost much because the condition number was large.

Example with R 9.17. To carry out the previous example in R, we restrict each factor in the SVD of the matrix B to just two columns and then multiply. The truncated pseudoinverse is computed similarly. Then we compute the approximate Moore–Penrose solution.

```
#truncated SVD/pseudoinverse
B=matrix(c(1,1,1,1,1,1,0,0,0,0,1,1,.05,-.05,.05,-.05),
    nrow=4)
p=matrix(c(1,3,8,2))
B0=svd(B)
##rank-2 truncated SVD
B2=B0$u[,1:2]%*%diag(B0$d[1:2])%*%t(B0$v[,1:2])
#truncated pseudoinverse
B2.plus=B0$v[,1:2]%*%diag(1/B0$d[1:2])%*%t(B0$u[,1:2])
##apply pseudoinverse to rhs vector
x2plus=B2.plus%*%p
```

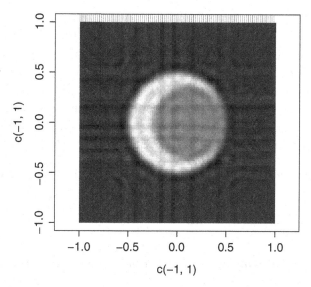

Fig. 9.4. This figure shows the image reconstruction from the truncated SVD of the coefficient matrix; the grid is $K \times K$ with $K = 100$ and 100 X-rays at each of 90 different angles. The largest $K\sqrt{K} = 1000$ singular values were used in the truncation.

To create an image from X-ray data using the truncated SVD, return to the system (9.6). Denoting the matrix of coefficients by A, the vector of unknown color values by $\mathbf{x}$, and the vector of scanner values by $\mathbf{p}$, the system we wish to solve is expressed as $A\mathbf{x} = \mathbf{p}$. The next step is to compute the singular value decomposition of the coefficient matrix A. Not surprisingly, for a realistic problem, this a huge computational effort. For the image in Figure 9.4, corresponding to an image grid with $K^2 = 100^2$ pixels and a scan involving 9090 X-ray lines, the SVD was truncated to the largest $K\sqrt{K} = 1000$ singular values. The corresponding modified pseudoinverse was then computed and applied to the vector of Radon transform values for a particular phantom. The resulting approximate Moore–Penrose solution gives us the vector of color values.

While the time needed to compute the SVD of the coefficient matrix for this system is substantial, the method is nonetheless quite versatile because the *same matrix can be used over and over again,* for every slice and for every scan of every patient. Thus, the only new computation each time is the last step of multiplying the truncated SVD by a new vector of right-hand sides. This step doesn't take much time at all. So we can get a lot of work out of that one big matrix factorization. By comparison, the filtered back-projection algorithm must be recomputed from scratch each time starting with the new Radon transform data from the latest scan.

Tikhonov regularization Truncating the singular value decomposition of the coefficient matrix is one way to manage the distortions introduced by using the pseudoinverse in the presence of zero or near-zero singular values. By restricting the computation, we can enforce an upper bound on the size of the reciprocals of the singular values being used.

A second approach to dealing with this problem is to modify the coefficient matrix so that all singular values are strictly positive. To see how we might accomplish this, consider again the equation $A\mathbf{x} = \mathbf{p}$. To compute the singular values, we look at the symmetric matrix $A^T A$ and its eigenvalue decomposition $A^T A = VDV^T$, where the columns of V form an orthonormal basis of eigenvectors of $A^T A$. The obstruction that concerns us here is that the matrix D might not be invertible. To remove this obstacle, take $\alpha > 0$ to be any strictly positive number, and let $D_1 = (D + \alpha^2 I)$, where I denotes the identity matrix of the appropriate size. The matrix D_1 is invertible, because it is a diagonal matrix with positive diagonal entries, all at least as big as α^2. We now compute $VD_1 V^T = A^T A + \alpha^2 I$, since $V^T = V^{-1}$. The matrix $A^T A + \alpha^2 I$ is symmetric, so $VD_1 V^T$ must be its eigenvalue decomposition. Next, let $A_1 = \begin{bmatrix} A \\ \alpha I \end{bmatrix}$ be the matrix formed when including the rows of αI below the rows of A. Thus, $A_1^T A_1 = [A^T\ \alpha I] \begin{bmatrix} A \\ \alpha I \end{bmatrix} = A^T A + \alpha^2 I$. Finally, form the vector $\mathbf{p}_1 = \begin{bmatrix} \mathbf{p} \\ 0 \end{bmatrix}$ by including the appropriate number of 0s below the coordinates of the vector $\mathbf{p}$. This gives us the computations $A_1^T A_1 \mathbf{x} = A^T A\mathbf{x} + \alpha^2 \mathbf{x}$ and $A_1^T \mathbf{p}_1 = A^T \mathbf{p}$. In other words, we can replace our original least squares problem, $A\mathbf{x} = \mathbf{p}$, with the new problem $A_1 \mathbf{x} = \mathbf{p}_1$, which has the corresponding normal equation $(A^T A + \alpha^2 I)\mathbf{x} = A_1^T \mathbf{p}_1$.

Thus, we are now interested in solving the minimization problem

$$\min_{\mathbf{x}} ||A_1 \mathbf{x} - \mathbf{p}_1||^2 = \min_{\mathbf{x}} \left\| \begin{bmatrix} A\mathbf{x} \\ \alpha\mathbf{x} \end{bmatrix} - \begin{bmatrix} \mathbf{p} \\ 0 \end{bmatrix} \right\|^2$$

$$= \min_{\mathbf{x}} \left\| \begin{bmatrix} A\mathbf{x} - \mathbf{p} \\ \alpha\mathbf{x} \end{bmatrix} \right\|^2$$

$$= \min_{\mathbf{x}} \left\{ ||A\mathbf{x} - \mathbf{p}||^2 + \alpha^2 ||\mathbf{x}||^2 \right\}, \qquad (9.15)$$

where the Pythagorean theorem gives us the last equality. This differs from the original problem in that we are no longer minimizing $||A\mathbf{x} - \mathbf{p}||^2$. Rather, we are willing to accept a larger value for this term if it means we can use a smaller $\mathbf{x}$ that reduces the value in (9.15).

Since the matrix $A_1^T A_1 = (A^T A + \alpha^2 I)$ is invertible, the normal equation for our new problem has an exact solution,

$$\mathbf{x}_\alpha = (A^T A + \alpha^2 I)^{-1} A^T \mathbf{p}. \qquad (9.16)$$

However, computing a matrix inverse can be perilous, due to round-off errors and other obstacles. So let's investigate the singular value decomposition approach to this problem.

Suppose we have the eigenvalue decomposition $A^T A = VDV^T$ and the corresponding singular value decomposition $A = U\Sigma V^T$, where $V^T = V^{-1}$ and $U^T = U^{-1}$, as before. Then $A_1^T A_1 = (A^T A + \alpha^2 I) = V(D + \alpha^2 I)V^T$. The matrix $(D + \alpha^2 I)$ is diagonal, with diagonal entries $\sigma_j^2 + \alpha^2$, where $\{\sigma_j\}$ are the singular values of A. The reciprocals of these numbers are the diagonal entries of the inverse matrix $(D + \alpha^2 I)^{-1}$.

For convenience, let $\Sigma_\alpha = (D + \alpha^2 I)^{-1} \Sigma^T$. To compute the solution $\mathbf{x}_\alpha$, given in (9.16), we need the matrix

$$\left(A^T A + \alpha^2 I\right)^{-1} A^T = \left(V(D + \alpha^2 I)^{-1} V^T\right)\left(V \Sigma^T U^T\right) = V \Sigma_\alpha U^T.$$

This is the pseudoinverse of a singular value decomposition. The diagonal entries of Σ_α are given by

$$\begin{cases} \frac{1}{\sigma_j}\left(\frac{\sigma_j^2}{\sigma_j^2 + \alpha^2}\right) & \text{if } \sigma_j > 0, \\ 0 & \text{if } \sigma_j = 0, \end{cases}$$

Notice that this is a sort of filtered form of the pseudoinverse $A^+ = V \Sigma^+ U^T$, in which the diagonal entries of Σ^+ are either $1/\sigma_j$ or 0, accordingly. In the matrix Σ_α, the nonzero entries have been damped by the factors $\sigma_j^2/(\sigma_j^2 + \alpha^2) < 1$. This damping reduces the distortion caused by large reciprocals $1/\sigma_j$.

Thus, the solution to the minimization problem (9.15) is

$$\mathbf{x}_\alpha = V \Sigma_\alpha U^T \mathbf{p} = \sum_{j:\sigma_j > 0} \frac{1}{\sigma_j}\left(\frac{\sigma_j^2}{\sigma_j^2 + \alpha^2}\right)\left(\mathbf{u}_j^T \mathbf{p}\right) \mathbf{v}_j. \tag{9.17}$$

Of course, we could truncate this sum if we wished to emphasize the contributions of the larger singular values.

Example 9.18. Once again, let $A = \begin{bmatrix} 1 & 1 & 0 \\ 1 & 1 & 0 \\ 1 & 0 & 1 \\ 1 & 0 & 1 \end{bmatrix}$ and $\mathbf{p} = (1, 3, 8, 2)$. For a first example, let's try $\alpha = 1$. The singular values of A are $\sqrt{6}$, $\sqrt{2}$, and 0. Thus, $\Sigma_\alpha = \begin{bmatrix} \frac{1}{\sqrt{6}}\left(\frac{6}{6+1}\right) & 0 & 0 & 0 \\ 0 & \frac{1}{\sqrt{2}}\left(\frac{2}{2+1}\right) & 0 & 0 \\ 0 & 0 & 0 & 0 \end{bmatrix}$. This yields the approximate solution $\mathbf{x}_\alpha = V \Sigma_\alpha U^T \mathbf{p} = $ (2, 0, 2). This is smoother than the Moore–Penrose solution, $\mathbf{x}^+ = (7/3, -1/3, 8/3)$, because the entries have been brought closer together. Looking at the normal equation, we get $A^T A \mathbf{x}_\alpha = (10, 4, 8)$, while $A^T \mathbf{p} = (14, 4, 10)$. This suggests that $\alpha = 1$ might be a bit large.

With $\alpha = 0.5$, we get $\Sigma_\alpha = \begin{bmatrix} \frac{1}{\sqrt{6}}\left(\frac{6}{6.25}\right) & 0 & 0 & 0 \\ 0 & \frac{1}{\sqrt{2}}\left(\frac{2}{2.25}\right) & 0 & 0 \\ 0 & 0 & 0 & 0 \end{bmatrix}$. This gives $\mathbf{x}_\alpha = $ (2.24, $-0.21\overline{33}$, $2.45\overline{33}$). This is much closer to the Moore–Penrose solution than our previous effort. Moreover, $A^T A \mathbf{x}_\alpha$ is also closer to $A^T \mathbf{p}$ than before. This suggests that $\alpha = 0.5$ may be a reasonable choice for the regularization parameter.

In the exercises, we will explore some other choices for α.

Example with R 9.19. Of course, we can do the previous example in *R*. A custom function, called `tik` here, computes the weighted diagonal elements.

```
A=matrix(c(1,1,1,1,1,1,0,0,0,0,1,1),nrow=4)
p=matrix(c(1,3,8,2))
A0=svd(A)
#select a regularization parameter;
#function "tik" to generate weights
tik=function(x,alpha){x/(x^2+alpha^2)}
w1=tik(A0$d,0.5)
#modified pseudoinverse
T1=round(A0$v%*%diag(w1)%*%t(A0$u),4)
#modified Moore--Penrose solution
xalpha=T1%*%p
t(A)%*%A%*%xalpha #(13.44, 4.0536, 9.3864)
```

In the context of tomography, we can apply the Tikhonov regularization method and formula (9.17) to the system of equations (9.6). As before, the solution is interpreted as a vector of color values for the pixels in the image grid. Figure 9.5 illustrates how the choice of the regularization parameter α affects the resulting image.

Remark 9.20. In Tikhonov regularization, the value of the parameter α is up to the user to choose. A very large value of α will damp the components of the solution too much; the resulting image will be over-smoothed. At the other extreme, choosing $\alpha = 0$ will bring us back to the Moore–Penrose solution and the image will be under-smoothed. Similarly, with the truncated SVD, if we use too few terms, the resulting image will not have enough detail; the image will be over-smoothed. But using too many terms will include too much distortion and noise, resulting in an under-smoothed image.

The so-called *damped least squares* or *generalized Tikhonov regularization* method involves selecting a matrix ϕ, which might approximate a derivative operator, for instance, and solving the minimization problem

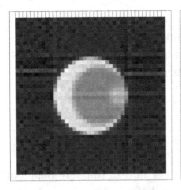 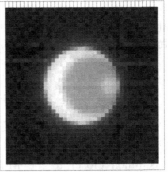 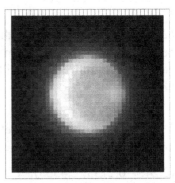

Fig. 9.5. Image reconstruction using ART and Tikhonov regularization. Left to right: $\alpha = 0.2$, $\alpha = 0.5$, and $\alpha = 1.0$.

$$\min_{\mathbf{x}} ||A\mathbf{x} - \mathbf{p}||^2 + \alpha^2 ||\Phi \mathbf{x}||^2 .$$

See [23] for more on this approach.

Remark 9.21. We have considered several approaches to finding approximate solutions to $A\mathbf{x} = \mathbf{p}$. In every case, our solution had the form $\sum \phi_j \frac{1}{\sigma_j} \left(\mathbf{u}_j^T \mathbf{p} \right) \mathbf{v}_j$, for some choice of weights $\{\phi_j\}$. For the Moore–Penrose solution, $\mathbf{x}^+$, we have $\phi_j = 1$ for all j. In the truncated SVD, ϕ_j has either the value 1, when j is small, or 0, when j is large. The solution $\mathbf{x}_\alpha$, produced by the Tikhonov regularization method, uses the weights $\phi_j = \left(\frac{\sigma_j^2}{\sigma_j^2 + \alpha^2} \right)$. A more general theory of *spectral filtering* allows for other choices of weights. We will not explore this any further here. See [37] or [23] for more information.

9.6 ART or the Fourier transform?

As mentioned at the start of this chapter, the first CT scanner, invented at EMI by Hounsfield, essentially used an ART approach for its images. However, Fourier transform methods, such as the filtered back-projection formula, are generally faster to implement on a computer. Consequently, today's commercial scanners are programmed to use transform methods. The iterative algorithms of ART simply converge too slowly, while the filtered back projection, which is based on a continuous model, can be adapted fairly easily to any desired level of accuracy.

It is nonetheless worth studying ART, and not only for its intrinsic mathematical interest. For instance, in some nonmedical applications of CT, such as nondestructive material testing, abrupt changes in the density of the material being scanned require image reconstruction methods that can provide high contrast. ART turns out to be useful in this regard. Also, ART can have a role to play in single-photon emission computerized tomography (SPECT) and positron emission tomography (PET), where difficulty in the measurement of the attenuation can sometimes render transform methods less reliable than usual. Finally, we mention the problem of incomplete data collection, which can occur, for instance, if the range of angles used in a CT scan is restricted in order to limit the patient's exposure to X-rays. Transform methods that rely on convolution require the completion of the data, whereas the iterative ART methods simply get applied to a smaller set of equations.

9.7 Exercises

1. For the system of two lines $x_1 - x_2 = 0$ and $x_1 + x_2 = 5$ and the starting point $\mathbf{x}^0 = \begin{bmatrix} 3 \\ 1 \end{bmatrix}$, apply Kaczmarz's method to compute $\mathbf{x}^{0,1}$ and $\mathbf{x}^{0,2}$. Show that the vector $\mathbf{x}^{0,2}$ lies on both lines.

2. For the system of three lines $x_1 - x_2 = 1$, $x_2 = 1$, and $x_1 = 0$ and the starting point $\mathbf{x}^0 = \begin{bmatrix} 0 \\ 0 \end{bmatrix}$, apply Kaczmarz's method to compute $\mathbf{x}^1$ and $\mathbf{x}^2$. (That is, apply two full cycles of the iteration.) What happens? What happens if we start instead at $\mathbf{x}^0 = \begin{bmatrix} a_1 \\ a_2 \end{bmatrix}$?

3. Prove Theorem B.7: Let A be an $M \times N$ matrix, let $\mathbf{x}$ be a vector in $\mathbb{R}^N$, and let $\mathbf{y}$ be a vector in $\mathbb{R}^M$. Then

$$Ax \bullet y = x \bullet A^T y .$$

4. Let A be an $M \times N$ matrix. Prove that, if $\mathbf{y}$ is in the nullspace of A^T, then $\mathbf{y}$ is orthogonal to the range of A. In conjunction with the Corollary B.8, this shows that the orthogonal complement of the range of A coincides with the nullspace of A^T.

5. Provide detailed solutions for Examples 9.10 and 9.11 in the text.

6. In each case, find all least squares solutions to the system $A\mathbf{x} = \mathbf{b}$.

   (a) $A = \begin{bmatrix} 4 & 0 \\ 0 & 2 \\ 1 & 1 \end{bmatrix}$; $\mathbf{b} = \begin{bmatrix} 2 \\ 0 \\ 11 \end{bmatrix}$.

   (b) $A = \begin{bmatrix} 1 & 1 & 0 & 0 \\ 1 & 1 & 0 & 0 \\ 1 & 0 & 1 & 0 \\ 1 & 0 & 1 & 0 \\ 1 & 0 & 0 & 1 \\ 1 & 0 & 0 & 1 \end{bmatrix}$; $\mathbf{b} = \begin{bmatrix} -3 \\ -1 \\ 0 \\ 2 \\ 5 \\ 1 \end{bmatrix}$. *Warning: $A^T A$ is not invertible!*

7. For a given $M \times N$ matrix A and a given vector $\mathbf{p}$ in $\mathbb{R}^M$, let the function $F : \mathbb{R}^N \to \mathbb{R}$ be defined by

$$F(\mathbf{x}) := ||A\mathbf{x} - \mathbf{p}||^2 = (A\mathbf{x} - \mathbf{p}) \bullet (A\mathbf{x} - \mathbf{p}) , \quad \text{for all } \mathbf{x} \text{ in } \mathbb{R}^N .$$

   Show that the *gradient vector* of F satisfies

$$\nabla F(\mathbf{x}) = 2 \left(A^T A \mathbf{x} - A^T \mathbf{p} \right) , \quad \text{for all } \mathbf{x} \text{ in } \mathbb{R}^N ,$$

   as claimed in (9.14).

8. Let $A = \begin{bmatrix} 1 & 2 \\ 1 & 2 \end{bmatrix}$ and $\mathbf{p} = \begin{bmatrix} 1 \\ 2 \end{bmatrix}$. Define F by

$$F(x, y) = \left\| A \begin{bmatrix} x \\ y \end{bmatrix} - \mathbf{p} \right\|^2.$$

By solving the equation $\nabla F(x, y) = \begin{bmatrix} 0 \\ 0 \end{bmatrix}$, show that the vector $\mathbf{q}$ in the range of A that is closest to $\mathbf{p}$ is $\mathbf{q} = \begin{bmatrix} 1.5 \\ 1.5 \end{bmatrix}$.

9. Verify the details of the solution to Example 9.12 in the text.

10. In Example 9.18, we used Tikhonov regularization, with the regularization parameters $\alpha = 1$ and $\alpha = 0.5$, to find approximate solutions to the system $A\mathbf{x} = \mathbf{p}$, where

$$A = \begin{bmatrix} 1 & 1 & 0 \\ 1 & 1 & 0 \\ 1 & 0 & 1 \\ 1 & 0 & 1 \end{bmatrix} \text{ and } \mathbf{p} = \begin{bmatrix} 1 \\ 3 \\ 8 \\ 2 \end{bmatrix}.$$

Now compute $\mathbf{x}_\alpha$ and $A^T A \mathbf{x}_\alpha$ for $\alpha = 2$ and $\alpha = 1/\sqrt{10}$ (so $\alpha^2 = 0.1$).

MRI — an overview

10.1 Introduction

Magnetic resonance imaging, or MRI, is an imaging technique that has grown alongside CT and that, like CT, has produced Nobel laureates of its own. Where the physics of CT is fairly straightforward — X-rays are emitted and their changes in intensity measured — MRI is based on the generation of a complex of overlapping, fluctuating electromagnetic fields that must be precisely controlled. Mathematically, the effects of the electromagnetic fields on the atomic nuclei in the sample being studied are modeled with differential equations. The Fourier transform is the primary tool for analyzing the electrical signals generated by the motions of atomic nuclei under the influence of these fields.

Clinically, MRI is safer than CT for most patients since it involves no radiation. The magnetic fields involved operate at frequencies in the radio band range. (In fact, to the patient undergoing an MRI exam, it sounds like listening to a very loud, very weird radio station.) In order to emphasize the safety and to discourage confusion, the original appellation of *nuclear magnetic resonance imaging* (nMRI) was shortened. On the downside, an MRI machine is expensive to purchase, operate, and maintain. Also, the intensity of the magnetic fields can rule out the procedure for some patients, including those with certain metallic implants.

Magnetic resonance imaging is a wide-ranging and continually developing field of study and practice, and is the subject of an extensive body of literature. Consequently, in this chapter we present only a brief overview of some of the basic principles involved in MRI, emphasizing aspects of the underlying mathematics. For a reader wishing to undertake a more intensive investigation of MRI, some possible starting points are the article [26] and the books [5, 20, 21], and [33].

Two basic descriptions of the phenomenon known as nuclear magnetic resonance (NMR) were published in 1946, one by a team of researchers led by Felix Bloch (1905–1983) and the other by a team headed by Edward Purcell (1912–1997). Bloch's point of view (see [4]) is based on principles from classical physics and adopts an aggregate approach, looking at

© Springer International Publishing Switzerland 2015
T.G. Feeman, *The Mathematics of Medical Imaging*, Springer Undergraduate
Texts in Mathematics and Technology, DOI 10.1007/978-3-319-22665-1_10

the net magnetization of the nuclei in a sample. Purcell's description ([41]) is grounded in quantum physics and examines the magnetic effects at the level of an individual nucleus. It is perhaps ironic that Bloch was trained as a quantum physicist (his doctoral advisor was Werner Heisenberg), while Purcell was a classical physicist (his doctoral advisor was John van Vleck). In 1952, Bloch and Purcell were joint recipients of the Nobel Prize for Physics.

For several decades after Bloch and Purcell established the physical basis for studying NMR, the primary application was to chemical spectroscopy, and it was only around 1970 that the possibility of using NMR for imaging was realized. Paul Lauterbur (1929–2007) is credited with introducing the idea of using gradient magnetic fields to achieve spatial resolution of the radio signal emitted by a magnetized sample. Applying his technology to a setup consisting of test tubes of heavy water sitting inside a beaker of regular water, he produced the first images that could distinguish between two different kinds of water. (See [34].) Peter Mansfield (1933 –) advanced Lauterbur's work by developing techniques for mathematically analyzing the radio signals, including a technique known as echo-planar imaging that speeds up the imaging process. (See [38].) Lauterbur and Mansfield were jointly awarded the 2003 Nobel Prize for Medicine and Physiology.

10.2 Basics

The nucleus of a hydrogen atom, a chemical element found in abundance in the human body, possesses a property known as spin. Conceptually, one can think of the single proton that comprises this nucleus as a tiny spinning top, rotating about an axis. This property brings with it a magnetic effect, whereby the spinning proton behaves like a bar magnet with north and south poles. As the little magnet spins, it generates an electrical signal. In the absence of other factors, there is no preferred choice for the axis around which the proton spins nor for the orientation of this axis within three-dimensional space. Within a sample of hydrogen-rich tissue, then, the distribution of spins will be random and the resulting signals will cancel each other out.

If, however, the sample is immersed in a strong external magnetic field having a fixed direction, then the spin axes of the hydrogen protons will tend to align either in the same direction as the external field or in the opposite direction. There will be some of each, but measurably more in the same direction as the field, as this state involves a lower energy level. To be more precise, the axes of the spinning hydrogen protons will not align exactly with the external field but will precess, or wobble, about it, much as a spinning top whose axis is not vertical precesses about the vertical as it spins. Due to the precession, the magnetic moment of any one particular nucleus will have a vector component that is perpendicular to the direction of the external field. However, because there is no preferred phase for the precession, the phases of the various nuclei in the sample will be randomly distributed and, as a result, the sum of these components will cancel out. Over the whole sample, then, the effect is of an aggregate nuclear magnetic moment that is aligned in the same direction as the external magnetic field.

In this equilibrium state, with all of the nuclei behaving in basically the same way, exhibiting a sort of herd mentality, no useful electrical signal will be generated. To create a signal, a second magnetic field is introduced, one that oscillates in a plane perpendicular to the static external field. This new field causes the alignment of the nuclei to flip out of the equilibrium state. As the nuclei begin to precess about a new axis, the specifics of which depend on the strength and duration of the new field, the aggregate nuclear magnetic moment develops a nonzero net component transverse to the static magnetic field. After a certain amount of time, this second field is cut off and the nuclei relax back to their previous state. There are two aspects to this relaxation.

As the net transverse component of the magnetic moment precesses, it induces an electromotive force (emf) in a coil that surrounds the sample. At the same time, with only the static field in effect, the nuclei gradually become de-phased in the transverse direction as they move toward equilibrium. Essentially, the net transverse magnetization describes a decaying wave, the rate of decay of which can be measured by analyzing the resulting induced emf. This process is known as *spin–spin*, or T_2, relaxation.

While the transverse component of the nuclear magnetic moment decays to zero, the component in the direction of the static magnetic field returns, asymptotically, to its equilibrium level. This process is called *spin–lattice*, or T_1, relaxation. As we shall see, the rate at which this process evolves can be measured through careful manipulation of the second magnetic field and the analysis of an electrical signal induced by the motion of the aggregate nuclear magnetic moment.

Different tissue types, or, more precisely, magnetized nuclei contained inside different chemical environments, have different T_1 and T_2 relaxation rates, the measurements of which reveal the types of material present within the sample. To resolve this information spatially, so that an image can be created showing the location within the sample of each type of tissue, additional magnetic fields, known as gradients, are introduced to the experiment. This is discussed in what follows.

At the molecular and atomic level, quantum effects certainly exist, but the classical approach outlined here is more feasible when it comes to designing practical machines to implement the system. So, with this conceptual framework in mind, we turn our attention to the mathematical model introduced by Bloch in 1946.

10.3   The Bloch equation

In an MRI machine, a strong, uniform, and steady magnetic field, $\mathbf{B}_0$, is generated by running an electrical current through a large coil. In clinical applications, the direction of the field $\mathbf{B}_0$ is aligned along the length of the patient's body, which direction is taken as the z-axis of a Cartesian coordinate system and is also referred to as the *longitudinal* direction. The magnitude or strength of $\mathbf{B}_0$, denoted by B_0 (without the boldface type), is usually about 0.5 tesla in practice.

Denote the aggregate magnetic moment of the nuclei in a sample by $\mathbf{M}(t, \mathbf{p})$, or simply by $\mathbf{M}$ if the context is understood. This is a vector function that depends both on time t and on the location $\mathbf{p}$ within the sample. The coordinate functions of $\mathbf{M}$ are denoted by $M_x, M_y,$ and M_z. That is, for each time t and each point $\mathbf{p}$ in the sample,

$$\mathbf{M}(t, \mathbf{p}) = \langle M_x(t, \mathbf{p}), M_y(t, \mathbf{p}), M_z(t, \mathbf{p}) \rangle.$$

As discussed above, in the presence of the static magnetic field $\mathbf{B}_0$ alone, the equilibrium nuclear magnetization of the sample is directed along the z-axis. That is, at equilibrium, $\mathbf{M} = \langle 0, 0, M_{eq} \rangle$, where M_{eq} is the magnitude of this vector.

In addition to the steady magnetic field $\mathbf{B}_0$, a variety of other magnetic fields are introduced. These additional fields alter the magnitude and alignment of the nuclear magnetization of the sample and vary both temporally and spatially. Here, we use $\mathbf{B} = \mathbf{B}(t, \mathbf{p})$ to denote the total external magnetic field experienced by the sample at time t and location $\mathbf{p}$.

The *Bloch equation* models the rate of change over time of the magnetic moment of the nuclei at each point in the sample. With the notation just introduced, the equation is

$$\frac{d\mathbf{M}}{dt} = \gamma \, \mathbf{M} \times \mathbf{B} - \frac{\langle M_x, M_y, 0 \rangle}{T_2} - \frac{\langle 0, 0, M_z - M_{eq} \rangle}{T_1}, \tag{10.1}$$

where γ, T_1, and T_2 are constants. For reasons that will be clear soon, the value of γ is related to the resonant frequency of the system, while T_1 and T_2 are called the *relaxation times*.

In the presence only of the static magnetic field $\mathbf{B}_0 = \langle 0, 0, B_0 \rangle$, directed along the z-axis, the Bloch equation simplifies to the system of equations

$$\frac{dM_x}{dt} = \gamma B_0 M_y(t) - \frac{M_x(t)}{T_2},$$

$$\frac{dM_y}{dt} = -\gamma B_0 M_x(t) - \frac{M_y(t)}{T_2},$$

$$\frac{dM_z}{dt} = -\frac{M_z(t) - M_{eq}}{T_1}. \tag{10.2}$$

The first two of these equations define a first-order linear system with a constant coefficient matrix that can be solved using standard eigenvalue–eigenvector methods. The third equation can be treated either as a separable equation or as a first order linear equation. The upshot of this analysis is that

$$M_x(t) = e^{-t/T_2} \left(M_x(0) \cos(\omega_0 t) - M_y(0) \sin(\omega_0 t) \right),$$

$$M_y(t) = e^{-t/T_2} \left(M_x(0) \sin(\omega_0 t) + M_y(0) \cos(\omega_0 t) \right), \text{ and}$$

$$M_z(t) = M_z(0)e^{-t/T_1} + M_{eq} \left(1 - e^{-t/T_1} \right), \tag{10.3}$$

where $\omega_0 = -\gamma B_0$. Thus, we see that, for times t that are large compared to the value of T_1, the longitudinal component $M_z(t)$ tends toward the equilibrium magnetization M_{eq}. Meanwhile, in the transverse plane, as the xy-plane is called in this context, the magnetic moment of the nuclei rotates, or precesses, about the z-axis with angular frequency $\omega_0 = -\gamma B_0$ radians per second, known as the *Larmor frequency*. The constant γ, called the *gyromagnetic ratio*, typically has a value of about 2.68×10^8 radians per second per tesla, or, equivalently, about 42.6 megahertz (MHz) per tesla. (One hertz is one cycle per second, or 2π radians per second.) Thus, in a typical MRI experiment, the Larmor frequency lies in the radio frequency band. In comparison, X-rays have a much higher frequency of about 3 gigahertz.

As $t \to \infty$, the transverse component of the nuclear magnetization tends to 0, which does not mean, however, that the precession of the individual nuclei about the z-axis ceases. Rather, these rotations go out of phase with each other so that the distribution of the individual moments becomes random and the aggregate transverse component tends to zero. In the equilibrium state, each nucleus tends to precess with angular frequency ω_0 about the z-axis with longitudinal component M_{eq}. A useful image, again, is that of a spinning top whose axis is not vertical but precesses about the vertical with a fixed frequency.

The constant T_1 is called the *spin–lattice* relaxation time and reflects the dissipation in energy away from the spinning nuclei (the spin system) as the atomic and molecular structure (the lattice) of the sample settles into the equilibrium state. The *spin–spin* relaxation time, as T_2 is known, reflects the randomization of the phases of the spinning nuclei as the aggregate transverse component goes to 0. Thus, T_2 reflects the dissipation of energy within the spin system.

10.4 The RF field

No signal is emitted by the atomic nuclei so long as they are subjected only to the static magnetic field $\mathbf{B}_0$. To knock them out of this equilibrium, a radio frequency (RF) transmitter is used to apply a linearly polarized RF magnetic field

$$\mathbf{B}_1 = \langle 2B_1 \cos(\omega t), 0, 0 \rangle.$$

This field is generated by sending an oscillating electrical current through a transmitting coil that surrounds the sample. The field $\mathbf{B}_1$ oscillates along the x-axis with frequency ω, called the *irradiation frequency*, and is effectively the sum of two circularly polarized fields that oscillate in the xy-plane with the same frequency but in opposite directions. Namely,

$$\mathbf{B}_1 = \langle B_1 \cos(\omega t), B_1 \sin(\omega t), 0 \rangle + \langle B_1 \cos(\omega t), -B_1 \sin(\omega t), 0 \rangle.$$

Physically, the nuclei, and, hence, the aggregate magnetic moment, are significantly affected only by the circular field that oscillates in the same direction as the precession. This means that we may take

$$\mathbf{B}_1 = \langle B_1 \cos(\omega t), B_1 \sin(\omega t), 0 \rangle \tag{10.4}$$

to be the effective RF magnetic field.

The magnetic field in the longitudinal direction consists of the static field $\mathbf{B}_0$ and the contribution from the gradient field, $\mathbf{B}_G$, discussed below. The overall magnetic field applied to the sample is, then,

$$\mathbf{B} = \mathbf{B}_1 + \mathbf{B}_0 + \mathbf{B}_G = \langle B_1 \cos(\omega t), B_1 \sin(\omega t), B_0 + B_G \rangle. \tag{10.5}$$

The duration of the RF pulse is short relative to the values of T_1 and T_2, sufficiently so that we may ignore the T_1 and T_2 terms when we analyze the Bloch equation (10.1) during this time interval. So, in this context, the Bloch equation leads to a system of linear differential equations with nonconstant coefficients; specifically,

$$\frac{dM_x}{dt} = \gamma(B_0 + B_G)M_y - \gamma B_1 M_z \sin(\omega t),$$

$$\frac{dM_y}{dt} = -\gamma(B_0 + B_G)M_x + \gamma M_z B_1 \cos(\omega t),$$

$$\frac{dM_z}{dt} = \gamma B_1 M_x \sin(\omega t) - \gamma B_1 M_y \cos(\omega t). \tag{10.6}$$

To render this system more amenable to solution, it is convenient to introduce a rotating coordinate frame for the transverse plane, rather than the usual x- and y-coordinates. To this end, let $\mathbf{e}_1 = \langle \cos(\omega t), \sin(\omega t) \rangle$ and $\mathbf{e}_2 = \langle -\sin(\omega t), \cos(\omega t) \rangle$, and set

$$u(t) = M_x(t) \cos(\omega t) + M_y(t) \sin(\omega t) \text{ and}$$

$$v(t) = M_y(t) \cos(\omega t) - M_x(t) \sin(\omega t). \tag{10.7}$$

Thus,

$$M_x = u \cos(\omega t) - v \sin(\omega t) \text{ and}$$

$$M_y = u \sin(\omega t) + v \cos(\omega t). \tag{10.8}$$

The vector $\langle M_x(t), M_y(t) \rangle$ in the standard coordinate frame is the same as the vector $u(t)\mathbf{e}_1 + v(t)\mathbf{e}_2$ in the rotating frame.

Translated into the rotating frame, (10.6) yields the system

$$\frac{du}{dt} = [\gamma(B_0 + B_G) + \omega]v,$$

$$\frac{dv}{dt} = -[\gamma(B_0 + B_G) + \omega]u + \gamma B_1 M_z,$$

$$\frac{dM_z}{dt} = -\gamma B_1 v. \tag{10.9}$$

Suppose now that the RF transmitter is set so that the irradiation frequency matches the Larmor frequency. That is, suppose that we set $\omega = \omega_0$. Then the RF magnetic field oscillates in resonance with the natural frequency of the nuclei in the presence of the static field. With the rotating reference frame rotating about the z-axis at the same frequency as that at which the nuclei precess about the z-axis, it appears, from the point of view of the nuclei themselves, that they are not precessing at all. In other words, the apparent effect is as if there were no static field. This is what is behind the use of the word *resonance* in the terms *nuclear magnetic resonance* and *magnetic resonance imaging*. To see how this affects the mathematical model, take $\omega = \omega_0 = -\gamma B_0$ in (10.9) to get the system

$$\frac{du}{dt} = \gamma B_G v \,,$$

$$\frac{dv}{dt} = -\gamma B_G u + \gamma B_1 M_z \,,$$

$$\frac{dM_z}{dt} = -\gamma B_1 v \,. \tag{10.10}$$

If, in addition, we set $B_G = 0$ and assume that B_1 is constant, then (10.10) has constant coefficients and its solution is

$$u(t) = u(0) \,,$$

$$v(t) = v(0) \cos(-\gamma B_1 t) - M_z(0) \sin(-\gamma B_1 t) \,, \text{ and}$$

$$M_z(t) = M_z(0) \cos(-\gamma B_1 t) + v(0) \sin(-\gamma B_1 t). \tag{10.11}$$

Thus, when viewed in the rotating coordinate frame, the aggregate magnetization vector of the nuclei in the sample precesses around the $\mathbf{e}_1$-axis with frequency $\omega_1 = -\gamma B_1$. Meanwhile, the $\mathbf{e}_1$-axis itself rotates around the z-axis at the Larmor frequency.

10.5   RF pulse sequences; T_1 and T_2

To generate a signal, suppose that the RF transmitter, whose irradiation frequency matches the Larmor frequency, is cut off after a time of τ seconds. The nuclear magnetic moment will then begin to relax from its state of precession about the $\mathbf{e}_1$-axis back towards its equilibrium state of precession about the z-axis. As mentioned before, the aggregate nuclear magnetic moment now has a nonzero component transverse to the static magnetic field. As this net transverse component of the magnetic moment relaxes, an emf is induced in a coil surrounding the sample.

For instance, suppose that the oscillating RF magnetic field is cut off after time τ_1, where $-\gamma B_1 \tau_1 = \pi/2$. This is called a $\pi/2$ pulse or a 90° pulse. From (10.11), we see that the net magnetization of the sample at time τ_1, when viewed in the rotating frame, is given by

$$u(\tau_1) = u(0) \,, \quad v(\tau_1) = -M_z(0) \,, \text{ and } M_z(\tau_1) = v(0). \tag{10.12}$$

That is, the effect of this RF field is that the orientation of the aggregate magnetization vector has been flipped by an angle of $\pi/2$, or $90°$, from alignment with the z-axis into alignment with the $\mathbf{e}_2$-axis.

A second important RF pulse is the π, or $180°$, pulse, in which an RF magnetic field, oscillating at the Larmor frequency, is cut off after time τ_2, with $-\gamma B_1 \tau_2 = \pi$. (Obviously, $\tau_2 = 2\tau_1$.) At the instant when the field is cut off, the net magnetization in the sample is

$$u(\tau_2) = u(0) \, , \; v(\tau_2) = -v(0) \, , \; \text{and } M_z(\tau_2) = -M_z(0). \tag{10.13}$$

Thus, the orientation of the aggregate magnetization vector has been flipped by an angle of π, or $180°$, from alignment with the positive z-axis into alignment with the negative z-axis.

In the *inversion recovery* method for measuring T_1, a $180°$ RF pulse is applied in order to align the aggregate nuclear magnetization with the negative z-axis. After the pulse has been cut off, a time τ is allowed to pass, during which the magnetization partially recovers back toward the equilibrium state. Then a $90°$ RF pulse is applied to flip the partially recovered magnetization into the xy-plane. Following this pulse, the resulting signal is acquired. The size of the signal depends on the value of $M_z(\tau)$. Once the signal has been acquired, the magnetization is allowed to relax all the way back to equilibrium.

From (10.3), we see that

$$(M_{eq} - M_z(\tau)) = (M_{eq} - M_z(0)) \, e^{-\tau/T_1}.$$

Hence,

$$\ln(M_{eq} - M_z(\tau)) = \ln(M_{eq} - M_z(0)) - \tau/T_1.$$

This means that, if we graph the value of $\ln(M_{eq} - M_z(\tau))$ against the value of τ, the result is a straight line of slope $-1/T_1$. The signal acquisition step tells us the value of $M_z(\tau)$, so, by applying the inversion recovery pulse sequence just described for a variety of values of τ, we can determine the value of T_1.

One technical detail is that, because the signals involved are fairly weak, the pulse sequence should be repeated several times for each selected value of τ in order to increase the signal-to-noise ratio, and thus our confidence, in the measurement of $M_z(\tau)$.

The inversion recovery method is typically abbreviated as

$$(180° - -\tau - -90° - -AT - -t_\infty)_n \, ,$$

where AT refers to the signal acquisition time and the value of t_∞ is large compared to T_1 so that the magnetization has time to relax back to equilibrium. (Generally, take $t_\infty > 4 \cdot T_1$.) The subscript n indicates the number of times the sequence is to be repeated for each selected value of τ.

Another approach to measuring T_1 is *saturation recovery*, abbreviated as

$$(90° - -HS - -\tau - -90° - -AT - -HS)_n \, .$$

In this scheme, *HS* refers to the application of a magnetic field pulse that destroys the homogeneity of the static magnetic field and results in a system that is saturated — the nuclear magnetic moments are scattered. After time τ, the magnetization has partially recovered back toward equilibrium. This magnetization is flipped into the *xy*-plane by a 90° pulse, and the resulting signal, which depends on $M_z(\tau)$, is measured. Then the field homogeneity is destroyed again and the sequence is repeated. As with inversion recovery, a semi-log plot of $\ln(M_{eq} - M_z(\tau))$ as a function of τ produces a straight line of slope $-1/T_1$.

The principal method for measuring the value of T_2 is called *spin-echo*. First proposed, in 1950, by Hahn, this method is abbreviated

$$(90° - -\tau - -180°)_n \, .$$

The initial 90° RF pulse flips the magnetization into the *xy*-plane. Once this pulse has ended, we would expect the magnetization to precess at the fixed frequency ω_0 as it relaxes back to equilibrium. This would mean a constant component of magnetization in the direction of the e_2-axis in the rotating frame. However, there is really a small spread of frequencies, at least partly because of slight inhomogeneity in the static field. Thus, after some time τ has passed, the nuclear moments have fanned out a bit, with the ones that are rotating faster getting ahead of the slower ones. Application of a 180° RF pulse has the effect of flipping this fan over in the *xy*-plane, so that the faster rotators are now *behind* the slower ones. Thus, after another time lapse of duration τ, the moments will come back together, forming an *echo* of the magnetization that existed immediately following the original 90° pulse. The echo is weaker than the original, though, because of the random nature of spin–spin relaxation, which cannot be refocused, or undone, by the echo. During the time interval of length 2τ, the amplitude of the transverse magnetization will have diminished, or relaxed, by a factor of $e^{-2\tau/T_2}$. By repeating the process, we increase the signal-to-noise ratio in the measurements.

A variation on the spin-echo method is to use a train of 180° RF pulses spaced at intervals of 2τ, with signal acquisition midway between successive pulses.

10.6 Gradients and slice selection

The work we have done so far provides the foundation for the methods of NMR spectroscopy. There, the investigator's aim is basically to create a graph of the spectrum of the signal generated by the nuclear magnetic moments in a sample as they respond to some specific RF pulse sequence. As we shall discuss below, the different frequency components present in the signal, and their corresponding amplitudes, provide information about the variety of relaxation times and, hence, the variety of chemical environments present in the sample. In this way, the investigator can analyze the chemical composition of the sample.

The insight that earned a Nobel Prize for Lauterbur was that, by introducing yet another carefully controlled component to the magnetic field, it is possible to restrict the fluctuation in the aggregate magnetic moment of the sample to a specified slice within the sample. In other words, it is possible to localize the behavior of the nuclear magnetic moments and thereby generate an image of a specified slice that reveals the locations of the various chemical environments to be found there. This is the core idea behind magnetic resonance imaging, or MRI. A typical MRI study consists of creating a whole series of such images that, collectively, help the investigator to form a sense of the three-dimensional composition and structure of a sample.

The key to slice selection is to introduce a magnetic field, $\mathbf{B}_G$, that is oriented in the same direction as the static external field but that varies in magnitude according to the location within the sample. To achieve this, $\mathbf{B}_G$ is actually composed of three separately controlled magnetic fields. The first of these three varies in magnitude in proportion to the x-coordinate of the point in the sample; the magnitude of the second field is proportional to the y-coordinate of the location; and the magnitude of the third field is proportional to the z-coordinate. That is, there are constants G_1, G_2, and G_3 such that, at the point $\mathbf{p} = \langle x, y, z \rangle$,

$$\mathbf{B}_G(\mathbf{p}) = \langle 0, 0, G_1 x + G_2 y + G_3 z \rangle$$
$$= \langle 0, 0, \mathbf{G} \bullet \mathbf{p} \rangle, \tag{10.14}$$

where $\mathbf{G} = \langle G_1, G_2, G_3 \rangle$. This magnetic field is called a *gradient field* because the constants G_1, G_2, and G_3 measure the gradient of the field as the location varies within the sample. The magnitude of $\mathbf{B}_G$ at the point $\mathbf{p}$ is $B_G(\mathbf{p}) = |\mathbf{G} \bullet \mathbf{p}|$.

Geometrically, the set $\{\mathbf{p} : \mathbf{G} \bullet \mathbf{p} = 0\}$ defines a plane through the origin with normal vector $\mathbf{G}$. Now, let

$$G = |\mathbf{G}| = \sqrt{G_1{}^2 + G_2{}^2 + G_3{}^2}$$

and observe that, for any given number $\alpha > 0$, the vector $\mathbf{r}_\alpha = (\alpha/G)\mathbf{G}$ satisfies $\mathbf{r}_\alpha \bullet \mathbf{G} = \alpha G$ and $|\mathbf{r}_\alpha| = \alpha$. Thus, the set

$$\{\mathbf{p} : |\mathbf{G} \bullet \mathbf{p}| \le \alpha G\} \tag{10.15}$$

defines a slice of thickness 2α centered at the origin and normal to $\mathbf{G}$. In this way, we can select a slice of the sample that we wish to image, identify an appropriate normal vector $\mathbf{G}$, and tailor the gradient magnetic field $\mathbf{B}_G$ accordingly. (Experimentally, it is possible to locate the origin at any desired point within the sample, so it suffices to consider slices centered on the origin.)

The total magnetic field is now given by (10.5) and the Bloch equation has the form given in (10.6). Taking $\omega = \omega_0 = -\gamma B_0$, the Larmor frequency, and viewing the system in the rotating frame (10.7), the Bloch equation translates into the system in (10.10). That is, we have

$$\frac{du}{dt} = \gamma B_G v,$$

$$\frac{dv}{dt} = -\gamma B_G u + \gamma B_1 M_z \, ,$$

$$\frac{dM_z}{dt} = -\gamma B_1 v \, . \tag{10.16}$$

The T_1 and T_2 terms are not present in this system, so we are assuming that the duration of the gradient magnetic field is short compared to the relaxation times. If we also assume that the RF field $\mathbf{B}_1$ is weak, then (10.16) yields $M_z(t) \approx M_z(0)$ and we can write the other two equations as

$$\frac{du}{dt} = \gamma B_G v = -\omega_G v \, ,$$

$$\frac{dv}{dt} = -\gamma B_G u + \gamma B_1 M_z(0) = \omega_G u + \gamma B_1 M_z(0) \, , \tag{10.17}$$

where $\omega_G = -\gamma B_G$.

Now introduce the complex-number-valued function

$$\phi(t) = u(t) + i \cdot v(t) \, . \tag{10.18}$$

Differentiating, and using (10.17), we get

$$\begin{aligned}
\frac{d\phi}{dt} &= \frac{du}{dt} + i \cdot \frac{dv}{dt} \\
&= -\omega_G v + i \cdot \omega_G u + i \cdot \gamma B_1 M_z(0) \\
&= i \cdot \omega_G \cdot \phi(t) + i \cdot B_1 M_z(0) \, .
\end{aligned} \tag{10.19}$$

This is a first-order linear differential equation with integrating factor $e^{-i\omega_G t}$. With the initial condition $\phi(0) = 0$, the solution is

$$\phi(t) = i\gamma M_z(0) e^{i\omega_G t} \cdot \left\{ \int_0^t B_1(s) \cdot e^{-i\omega_G s} \, ds \right\} \, . \tag{10.20}$$

Substituting $\omega_G = -\gamma B_G = -\gamma (\mathbf{G} \bullet \mathbf{p})$ into (10.20) gives us

$$\phi(t, \mathbf{p}) = i\gamma M_z(0) e^{-i\gamma (\mathbf{G} \bullet \mathbf{p})t} \cdot \left\{ \int_0^t B_1(s) \cdot e^{i\gamma (\mathbf{G} \bullet \mathbf{p})s} \, ds \right\} \, . \tag{10.21}$$

Next, note that the RF pulse is exactly that — a pulse. So it shuts off after a certain amount of time τ. Thus, $B_1(s) = 0$ for $s \le 0$ and for $s > \tau$. It follows that $\phi(t, \mathbf{p}) = \phi(\tau, \mathbf{p})$ for all $t > \tau$. Using (10.21) and a change of variables in the integration, we see that, for $t > \tau$,

$$\phi(t, \mathbf{p}) = i\gamma M_z(0) e^{-i\gamma (\mathbf{G} \bullet \mathbf{p})\tau} \cdot \left\{ \int_0^\tau B_1(s) \cdot e^{i\gamma (\mathbf{G} \bullet \mathbf{p})s} \, ds \right\} \tag{10.22}$$

$$= i\gamma M_z(0)e^{-i\gamma(\mathbf{G}\bullet\mathbf{p})\tau} \cdot \left\{ \int_{s=-\tau/2}^{\tau/2} B_1(s+\tau/2) \cdot e^{i\gamma(\mathbf{G}\bullet\mathbf{p})(s+\tau/2)} \, ds \right\}$$

$$= i\gamma M_z(0)e^{-i\gamma(\mathbf{G}\bullet\mathbf{p})\tau/2} \cdot \left\{ \int_{s=-\tau/2}^{\tau/2} B_1(s+\tau/2) \cdot e^{i\gamma(\mathbf{G}\bullet\mathbf{p})s} \, ds \right\} .$$

Moreover, it follows from (10.22) that

$$|\phi(t, \mathbf{p})| = \gamma \, |M_z(0)| \cdot \left| \int_{s=-\tau/2}^{\tau/2} B_1(s+\tau/2) \cdot e^{i\gamma(\mathbf{G}\bullet\mathbf{p})s} \, ds \right| . \tag{10.23}$$

The integral in (10.22) and (10.23) is approximately equal to the inverse Fourier transform of the function $B_1(s+\tau/2)$ evaluated at $\gamma(\mathbf{G}\bullet\mathbf{p})$, provided that the value of $B_1(s+\tau/2)$ is small when $|s| > \tau/2$. In particular, if B_1 is a Gaussian, then the inverse Fourier transform of B_1 is also a Gaussian (see (5.22)). Hence, from (10.23), $|\phi(t, \mathbf{p})|$ will be large when $|\mathbf{G}\bullet\mathbf{p}|$ is small and, just as importantly, $|\phi(t, \mathbf{p})|$ will be small when $|\mathbf{G}\bullet\mathbf{p}|$ is large.

Specifically, consider the slice of thickness 2α defined, as in (10.15), by $\{\mathbf{p} : |\mathbf{G}\bullet\mathbf{p}| \leq \alpha G\}$. Shaping the RF pulse so that

$$B_1(s+\tau/2) = e^{-(\alpha\gamma Gs)^2/8} \tag{10.24}$$

results in

$$|\phi(t, \mathbf{p})| \text{ proportional to } e^{-2\left(\frac{\mathbf{G}\bullet\mathbf{p}}{\alpha\cdot G}\right)^2} . \tag{10.25}$$

Since $\int_{-1}^{1} e^{-2x^2} \, dx \approx 0.9545 \cdot \int_{-\infty}^{\infty} e^{-2x^2} \, dx$, the Gaussian in (10.25) has about 95% of its area in the selected slice. Hence, the transverse nuclear magnetic moment, as measured by $|\phi(t, \mathbf{p})|$, is predominantly concentrated in that slice.

10.7   The imaging equation

Having explored how an array of magnetic fields can be carefully orchestrated to produce a spatially encoded fluctuation in the transverse component of the nuclear magnetic moment of a sample, we will examine now, in only the coarsest fashion, how this leads to an image that is clinically useful.

The fluctuating magnetization of the nuclei in the sample induces an electromotive force (emf) in a coil surrounding the sample. Faraday's law of induction shows how to express this induced emf in terms of the derivative of the magnetization. In practice, it is most convenient to represent the magnetization in the sample by the complex-number-valued function

$$M^*(t, \mathbf{p}) = M_x(t, \mathbf{p}) + i \cdot M_y(t, \mathbf{p}) . \tag{10.26}$$

It follows from (10.7) and (10.18), that

$$\begin{aligned}
\left| M^*(t, \mathbf{p}) \right|^2 &= (M_x(t, \mathbf{p}))^2 + \left(M_y(t, \mathbf{p}) \right)^2 \\
&= (u(t, \mathbf{p}))^2 + (v(t, \mathbf{p}))^2 \\
&= |\phi(t, \mathbf{p})|^2 .
\end{aligned}$$

Thus, in the presence of the gradient magnetic field $\mathbf{B}_G$, the value of M^* is large inside the selected slice and small outside the slice.

The signal that is induced in the coil is sent through a preamplifier and then is subjected to a variety of treatments, including a phase detection step that shifts the signal down in frequency by ω_0 so that the frequencies present in the modified signal are centered around 0. This modification simplifies the signal analysis in later steps. Application of a low-pass filter increases the signal-to-noise ratio. At this stage, the signal $S(t)$, induced by the nuclear magnetization and modified by the receiver system, can be represented as

$$S(t) = K \int M^*(t, \mathbf{p}) \exp(-i\omega t) \, d\mathbf{p} , \tag{10.27}$$

where K is some complex number constant. This formula is called the *imaging equation*. It expresses the signal $S(t)$ as the (2- or 3-dimensional) Fourier transform of the complex transverse magnetization M^* of the sample. Thus, the function M^* can be recovered, and an image of it created, by applying the inverse Fourier transform.

In practice, the signal is sampled at a discrete set of times $\{k \cdot \Delta t\}$ and the inversion is done on a digital computer. Thus, some of the techniques discussed in Chapter 8 come into play, including sampling, the discrete Fourier transform and its inverse, and the fast Fourier transform.

10.8 Exercises

1. Verify that (10.3) is the solution to the system (10.2).
2. Verify that the system (10.6) is equivalent to the system (10.9) when translated into the rotating coordinate frame for the transverse plane.
3. Verify that (10.11) gives the solution to the system (10.10).
4. Verify that (10.20) is the solution to the system (10.19).

Appendix A

Integrability

A.1 Improper integrals

The Radon transform, back projection, and Fourier transform all involve *improper integrals*, evaluated over infinite intervals. We have applied these concepts, computing examples and proving theorems, without considering the more technical questions of how these improper integrals are defined and for what functions they make sense. We ought not evade these questions completely, so let us now attend to them.

Consider a function f, defined on the real line and having either real or complex values, with the property that the integral $\int_a^b f(x)\,dx$ exists for every finite interval $[a, b]$. If the limit $\lim_{b \to \infty} \int_a^b f(x)\,dx$ exists, then we denote this limit by $\int_a^\infty f(x)\,dx$ and we say that this improper integral converges. That is,

$$\int_a^\infty f(x)\,dx = \lim_{b \to \infty} \int_a^b f(x)\,dx$$

provided the limit exists.

Similarly,

$$\int_{-\infty}^b f(x)\,dx = \lim_{a \to -\infty} \int_a^b f(x)\,dx$$

provided the limit exists, in which case we say that the improper integral $\int_{-\infty}^b f(x)\,dx$ converges.

© Springer International Publishing Switzerland 2015
T.G. Feeman, *The Mathematics of Medical Imaging*, Springer Undergraduate
Texts in Mathematics and Technology, DOI 10.1007/978-3-319-22665-1

If both of the improper integrals $\int_a^\infty f(x)\,dx$ and $\int_{-\infty}^a f(x)\,dx$ converge for some real number a, then we define

$$\int_{-\infty}^\infty f(x)\,dx = \int_{-\infty}^a f(x)\,dx + \int_a^\infty f(x)\,dx.$$

Again we say that the improper integral $\int_{-\infty}^\infty f(x)\,dx$ converges and the function f is said to be *integrable* on the real line. If $|f|$ is integrable on the real line, then we say that f is *absolutely integrable*.

Some facts about improper integrals are similar to facts about infinite series. Here are a few, with the proofs left as exercises.

- If f and g are both integrable on $[a, \infty)$ and if c is any number, then $f + cg$ is also integrable on $[a, \infty)$ and

$$\int_a^\infty (f + cg)(x)\,dx = \int_a^\infty f(x)\,dx + c \int_a^\infty g(x)\,dx.$$

- If $f \geq 0$ and the set $\mathcal{S} = \{\int_a^b f(x)\,dx \,:\, b \geq a\}$ is bounded above, then $\int_a^\infty f(x)\,dx$ converges to the least upper bound of the set $\mathcal{S}$.
- If $|f(x)| \leq g(x)$ for all real x and the integral $\int_a^\infty g(x)\,dx$ converges, then $\int_a^\infty f(x)\,dx$ also converges and $\left|\int_a^\infty f(x)\,dx\right| \leq \int_a^\infty g(x)\,dx$. (This is a form of the comparison test. To prove it for f real-valued, apply the previous facts to $f = f_+ - f_-$, where $f_+(x) = \max\{f(x), 0\}$ and $f_-(x) = -\min\{f(x), 0\}$.)
- If $\int_a^\infty |f(x)|\,dx$ converges, then so does $\int_a^\infty f(x)\,dx$. In words, if f is absolutely integrable on $[a, \infty)$, then f is integrable there. This is a corollary of the previous fact. The converse statement is not true.

Similar statements prevail regarding improper integrals on $(-\infty, b)$ or on $(-\infty, \infty)$.

One large class of functions to which we can look for examples are the piecewise continuous functions. A real- or complex-valued function f, defined on the real line, is *piecewise continuous* if, in every finite interval $[a, b]$, there are only a finite number of points at which f is discontinuous and if the one-sided limits $\lim_{x \to a-} f(x)$ and $\lim_{x \to a+} f(x)$ both exist at each point of discontinuity α. Hence, we see that a piecewise continuous function is integrable on every finite interval of the real line. This is the starting point for asking whether any of the improper integrals above converge. The class of piecewise continuous functions will be denoted by $\mathcal{PC}$. This class includes all functions that are continuous on the real line.

Lebesgue's theory of integration makes it possible to extend the notion of integrability on the real line to more functions than the piecewise continuous ones. We will not go into this far-reaching theory here, but we will borrow the notation L^1 to denote the class of all (Lebesgue integrable) functions that are absolutely integrable on the real line. Thus, for instance, the set of piecewise continuous functions that are absolutely integrable is denoted by $L^1 \cap \mathcal{PC}$.

Since $|f(x)\,e^{-i\omega x}| = |f(x)|$ for all real numbers x and ω, it follows from the above facts that every function in L^1 has a Fourier transform. The Fourier inversion theorem (Theorem 5.12), however, applies only to continuous functions in L^1, though a modified version of it applies to functions in $L^1 \cap \mathcal{PC}$. This is ample motivation for restricting our attention mainly to functions in $L^1 \cap \mathcal{PC}$.

A.2 Iterated improper integrals

Another technical matter is the manipulation of iterated improper integrals over the plane. This shows up in the proof of the Fourier Inversion Theorem (Theorem 5.12), for instance, where the order of integration with respect to the two variables is switched in the middle of the proof. This begs the question of whether such a step is justified.

Suppose that g is a continuous function of two real variables such that, for some real number a, the improper integral $\int_a^\infty g(x, y)\,dx$ converges for every value of y in some interval $J = [\alpha, \beta]$. Then we say that this improper integral converges *uniformly* on J provided that, for every $\varepsilon > 0$, there exists a number B such that

$$\left| \int_a^b g(x, y)\,dx - \int_a^\infty g(x, y)\,dx \right| < \varepsilon \tag{A.1}$$

for all $b > B$ and all $y \in J$.

The relevant facts, found in standard texts in elementary real analysis (such as [2], for example), are these.

(i) With g as in the preceding paragraph, if $\int_a^\infty g(x, y)\,dx$ converges uniformly on the interval J, then the integral is a continuous function of y on J.

Proof. For each natural number n, let $G_n(y) = \int_a^{a+n} g(x, y)\,dx$. Each function G_n is continuous on J and the sequence $\{G_n\}$ converges uniformly on J to the function $G(y) = \int_a^\infty g(x, y)\,dx$. Hence, the function G is also continuous on J.   □

(ii) Again supposing g to be a continuous function of two real variables, if the integral $\int_a^\infty g(x, y)\,dx$ converges uniformly on the interval $J = [\alpha, \beta]$, then the improper integral $\int_a^\infty \int_\alpha^\beta g(x, y)\,dy\,dx$ converges and

$$\int_a^\infty \int_\alpha^\beta g(x, y)\,dy\,dx = \int_\alpha^\beta \int_a^\infty g(x, y)\,dx\,dy.$$

Proof. With G_n and G as defined in the preceding proof, the uniform convergence implies that

$$\int_\alpha^\beta G(y)\,dy = \lim_{n\to\infty} \int_\alpha^\beta G_n(y)\,dy.$$

That is,

$$\int_\alpha^\beta \int_a^\infty g(x,y)\,dx\,dy = \lim_{n\to\infty} \int_\alpha^\beta \int_a^{a+n} g(x,y)\,dx\,dy.$$

The continuity of g implies that iterated integrals over finite rectangles can be evaluated in either order, so that

$$\int_\alpha^\beta \int_a^{a+n} g(x,y)\,dx\,dy = \int_a^{a+n} \int_\alpha^\beta g(x,y)\,dy\,dx.$$

Hence,

$$\lim_{n\to\infty} \int_\alpha^\beta \int_a^{a+n} g(x,y)\,dx\,dy = \int_a^\infty \int_\alpha^\beta g(x,y)\,dy\,dx$$

and the desired result follows.   □

(iii) If g is continuous for $x \geq a$ and $y \geq \alpha$, and if the improper integrals $\int_a^\infty |g(x,y)|\,dx$ and $\int_\alpha^\infty |g(x,y)|\,dy$ converge uniformly on every finite interval, then if either of the integrals $\int_a^\infty \int_\alpha^\infty |g(x,y)|\,dy\,dx$ or $\int_\alpha^\infty \int_a^\infty |g(x,y)|\,dx\,dy$ converges,

$$\int_a^\infty \int_\alpha^\infty g(x,y)\,dy\,dx = \int_\alpha^\infty \int_a^\infty g(x,y)\,dx\,dy.$$

Proof. Suppose that $g \geq 0$ and that the integral $\int_\alpha^\infty \int_a^\infty g(x,y)\,dx\,dy$ converges. It follows from the previous result and the nonnegativity of g that, for each $b > a$,

$$\int_a^b \int_\alpha^\infty g(x,y)\,dy\,dx = \int_\alpha^\infty \int_a^b g(x,y)\,dx\,dy$$

$$\leq \int_\alpha^\infty \int_a^\infty g(x,y)\,dx\,dy.$$

Hence, $\int_a^\infty \int_\alpha^\infty g(x,y)\,dy\,dx$ converges by the comparison test, and

$$\int_a^\infty \int_\alpha^\infty g(x,y)\,dy\,dx \leq \int_\alpha^\infty \int_a^\infty g(x,y)\,dx\,dy.$$

Reversing the above argument shows that

$$\int_a^\infty \int_\alpha^\infty g(x,\ y)\,dy\,dx \geq \int_\alpha^\infty \int_a^\infty g(x,\ y)\,dx\,dy,$$

from which it follows that the integrals are equal, as claimed.

In general, for a real- or complex-valued function g that satisfies the hypotheses, we may write $g = g_1 - g_2 + ig_3 - ig_4$, where each of the functions g_j satisfies $0 \leq g_j \leq |g|$. (For instance, take $g_1(x,\ y) = \max\{\Re g(x, y),\ 0\}$.) The result then applies to each g_j and, by the linearity of the integral, to g itself.   □

A.3 L^1 and L^2

A function f defined on the real line is in the class L^2, and is said to be *square-integrable*, if the (improper) integral $\int_{-\infty}^\infty |f(x)|^2\,dx$ is finite. Neither L^1 nor L^2 is a subset of the other. For instance, the function f given by

$$f(x) = \begin{cases} 1/x \text{ if } x \geq 1, \\ 0 \ \ \text{ if } x < 1 \end{cases}$$

is in L^2 but not in L^1, while the function g defined by

$$g(x) = \begin{cases} 1/\sqrt{x} \text{ if } 0 < x \leq 1, \\ 0 \ \ \ \ \text{ otherwise} \end{cases}$$

is in L^1 but not in L^2.

The Rayleigh–Plancherel theorem (Theorem 7.11) applies to any absolutely integrable function f for which either f or its Fourier transform $\mathcal{F}f$ is square-integrable. In particular, for f in $L^1 \cap L^2$, it follows from (7.15) that $\mathcal{F}f$ is in L^2. Moreover, the mapping $f \mapsto \mathcal{F}f$ is an *isometry* from $L^1 \cap L^2$ into L^2.

It is a fact that $L^1 \cap L^2$ is dense in L^2 in the sense that, for every function f in L^2, there exists a sequence of functions $\{f_k\}$ in $L^1 \cap L^2$ such that

$$\lim_{k \to \infty} \int_{-\infty}^\infty |f(x) - f_k(x)|^2\,dx = 0.$$

(For instance, one may take f_k to be the restriction of f to the interval $[-k,\ k]$.) Each of the Fourier transforms $\mathcal{F}f_k$ is a well-defined function in L^2, and we may therefore define the Fourier transform of f to be the limit of the transforms $\mathcal{F}f_k$. (This limit exists because of the isometry implied by (7.15) and the fact that the space L^2 is complete.)

A modified form of the Fourier inversion theorem (Theorem 5.12) also holds in the L^2 setting so that, in the end, the mapping $f \mapsto \mathcal{F}f$ defines an isometric mapping from L^2 onto L^2. See Chapter 9 of [46] for a more in-depth discussion of these ideas.

A.4 Summability

Just as the Fourier transform and many of the theorems and computations accompanying it required the manipulation of improper integrals, so working with the discrete version of the Fourier transform can, in principle, involve working with infinite series and iterated infinite series. In practice, however, the discrete functions we use are always finite lists and the important theorems, like (8.22) and (8.24) to name two, use only finite sums.

The study of infinite series, Fourier series, and sequence spaces such as ℓ^1 and ℓ^2 is well worth the investment, but lies beyond the scope of our work here. The books [2] and [47] are good places to start.

Appendix B

Matrices, transposes, and factorization

In this appendix, we collect some results about matrices and their transposes. We also discuss two important matrix factorizations: the eigenvalue decomposition of a (real) symmetric matrix of the form $A^T A$ and the singular value decomposition of an arbitrary matrix. These basic tools are employed in our analysis of least squares approximation and in the image reconstruction techniques studied in Chapter 9. See the articles [29] and [50] and the texts [51] and [40] for more information, including additional applications of these concepts.

B.1 Transpose of a matrix

Definition B.1. For a given $M \times N$ matrix A, the *range* of A is the set $\{A\mathbf{x} \mid \mathbf{x} \in \mathbb{R}^N\}$. The *nullspace* of A is the set $\{\mathbf{x} \in \mathbb{R}^N \mid A\mathbf{x} = \mathbf{0}\}$. Notice that the range of A is a subset of $\mathbb{R}^M$, while the nullspace of A is a subset of $\mathbb{R}^N$.

Theorem B.2. *For a given $M \times N$ matrix A, the range of A is a subspace of $\mathbb{R}^M$ and the nullspace of A is a subspace of $\mathbb{R}^N$.*

Proof. If $\mathbf{x}_1$ and $\mathbf{x}_2$ are any elements of $\mathbb{R}^N$ and λ is any real constant (scalar), then

$$\lambda A\mathbf{x}_1 + A\mathbf{x}_2 = A(\lambda \mathbf{x}_1 + \mathbf{x}_2),$$

by the properties of matrix arithmetic. Thus, the range of A is closed under the operations of vector addition and scalar multiplication.

© Springer International Publishing Switzerland 2015
T.G. Feeman, *The Mathematics of Medical Imaging*, Springer Undergraduate
Texts in Mathematics and Technology, DOI 10.1007/978-3-319-22665-1

For the other claim, suppose $\mathbf{x}_1$ and $\mathbf{x}_2$ are elements of $\mathbb{R}^N$ such that $A\mathbf{x}_1 = A\mathbf{x}_2 = \mathbf{0}$, and let λ be any real number. Then

$$A(\lambda \mathbf{x}_1 + \mathbf{x}_2) = \lambda A\mathbf{x}_1 + A\mathbf{x}_2 = \lambda \cdot \mathbf{0} + \mathbf{0} = \mathbf{0}.$$

Thus, the nullspace of A is closed under the operations of vector addition and scalar multiplication. $\square$

Definition B.3. For a given $M \times N$ matrix A, the *transpose* of A, denoted by A^T, is the $N \times M$ matrix whose entry in row k and column j is the same as the entry of A in row j and column k. In other words, column j of A^T is the same as row j of A, and row k of A^T is the same as column k of A. Notice that, in general, $\left(A^T\right)^T = A$.

Example B.4. If $A = \begin{bmatrix} 4 & 0 \\ -3 & 2 \\ 1 & 5 \end{bmatrix}$, then $A^T = \begin{bmatrix} 4 & -3 & 1 \\ 0 & 2 & 5 \end{bmatrix}$.

Proposition B.5. *Let A be an $M \times N$ matrix and let B be an $N \times M$ matrix. Then*

$$(AB)^T = B^T A^T. \tag{B.1}$$

Proof. Notice that both matrices $(AB)^T$ and $B^T A^T$ are defined and have the same dimensions, $M \times M$. To see that these are indeed the same matrix, suppose A has entries $(a_{i,j})$ and that B has entries $(b_{i,j})$. Then the entry in row k and column j of both $(AB)^T$ and $B^T A^T$ is given by $\sum_{l=1}^{N} a_{j,l} \cdot b_{l,k}$. $\square$

Corollary B.6. *For any given $M \times N$ matrix A, the matrix $A^T A$ is equal to its own transpose. (Such a matrix is said to be symmetric.)*

The interaction between A, A^T, and the dot product, stated in the next theorem, is of fundamental importance in many applications of linear algebra.

Theorem B.7. *Let A be an $M \times N$ matrix, let $\mathbf{x}$ be a vector in $\mathbb{R}^N$, and let $\mathbf{y}$ be a vector in $\mathbb{R}^M$. Then*

$$A\mathbf{x} \bullet \mathbf{y} = \mathbf{x} \bullet A^T \mathbf{y}. \tag{B.2}$$

Notice that the dot product on the left-hand side involves two vectors in $\mathbb{R}^M$ while the dot product on the right-hand side involves two vectors in $\mathbb{R}^N$.

Proof. Let us consider an example to illustrate. Take $A = \begin{bmatrix} 4 & 0 \\ -3 & 2 \\ 1 & 5 \end{bmatrix}$, $\mathbf{x} = \begin{bmatrix} x_1 \\ x_2 \end{bmatrix}$ in $\mathbb{R}^2$, and

$\mathbf{y} = \begin{bmatrix} y_1 \\ y_2 \\ y_3 \end{bmatrix}$ in $\mathbb{R}^3$. Then we compute:

$$
\begin{aligned}
A\mathbf{x} \bullet \mathbf{y} &= \begin{bmatrix} 4 & 0 \\ -3 & 2 \\ 1 & 5 \end{bmatrix} \begin{bmatrix} x_1 \\ x_2 \end{bmatrix} \bullet \begin{bmatrix} y_1 \\ y_2 \\ y_3 \end{bmatrix} \\
&= \begin{bmatrix} 4x_1 \\ -3x_1 + 2x_2 \\ x_1 + 5x_2 \end{bmatrix} \bullet \begin{bmatrix} y_1 \\ y_2 \\ y_3 \end{bmatrix} \\
&= 4x_1 y_1 + (-3x_1 + 2x_2)y_2 + (x_1 + 5x_2)y_3 \\
&= x_1(4y_1 - 3y_2 + y_3) + x_2(2y_2 + 5y_3) \\
&= \begin{bmatrix} x_1 \\ x_2 \end{bmatrix} \bullet \begin{bmatrix} 4y_1 - 3y_2 + y_3 \\ 2y_2 + 5y_3 \end{bmatrix} \\
&= \begin{bmatrix} x_1 \\ x_2 \end{bmatrix} \bullet \begin{bmatrix} 4 & -3 & 1 \\ 0 & 2 & 5 \end{bmatrix} \begin{bmatrix} y_1 \\ y_2 \\ y_3 \end{bmatrix} \\
&= \mathbf{x} \bullet A^T \mathbf{y} \quad \text{as desired.}
\end{aligned}
$$

The general proof follows this same pattern and is left as an exercise.   □

Corollary B.8. *If* $\mathbf{y}$ *is orthogonal to the range of* A*, then* $\mathbf{y}$ *is in the nullspace of* A^T.

Proof. If $\mathbf{y}$ is orthogonal to the range of A, then $A\mathbf{x} \bullet \mathbf{y} = 0$ for every vector $\mathbf{x}$ in $\mathbb{R}^N$. Hence, it follows from Theorem B.7 that $\mathbf{x} \bullet A^T \mathbf{y} = 0$ for every $\mathbf{x}$ in $\mathbb{R}^N$. In other words, the vector $A^T \mathbf{y}$ is orthogonal to *every* vector in $\mathbb{R}^N$. In particular, the vector $A^T \mathbf{y}$ is *orthogonal to itself*, so that $A^T \mathbf{y} \bullet A^T \mathbf{y} = 0$. That is, $||A^T \mathbf{y}||^2 = 0$, from which it follows that $A^T \mathbf{y} = 0$. In other words, $\mathbf{y}$ is in the nullspace of A^T as claimed.   □

Theorem B.9. *For any matrix A, the nullspace of A is the same as the nullspace of $A^T A$.*

Proof. Let A be any matrix. Suppose $\mathbf{x}$ is in the nullspace of A, so that $A\mathbf{x} = \mathbf{0}$. Then, $A^T A\mathbf{x} = A^T \mathbf{0} = \mathbf{0}$, as well.

Conversely, suppose that $\mathbf{x}$ is in the nullspace of $A^T A$, so that $A^T A \mathbf{x} = \mathbf{0}$. Then, using Theorem B.2, we see that

$$||A\mathbf{x}||^2 = A\mathbf{x} \bullet A\mathbf{x} = \mathbf{x} \bullet A^T A \mathbf{x} = \mathbf{x} \bullet \mathbf{0} = 0. \tag{B.3}$$

Hence, $A\mathbf{x} = \mathbf{0}$, as well.

Thus, the matrices A and $A^T A$ have the same nullspace, as claimed. $\square$

B.2 Eigenvalue decomposition

We now turn to the eigenvalue decomposition of the symmetric matrix $A^T A$. Recall that a nonzero vector $\mathbf{v}$ in $\mathbb{R}^N$ is said to be an *eigenvector* of the $N \times N$ matrix B if there is a number λ for which $B\mathbf{v} = \lambda \mathbf{v}$. The number λ is called an *eigenvalue* of B.

Theorem B.10. *Let A be an $M \times N$ real matrix.*

(i)   *All eigenvalues of $A^T A$ are non-negative (real) numbers.*
(ii)   *Eigenvectors corresponding to different eigenvalues are orthogonal.*
(iii) *There is an orthonormal basis of $\mathbb{R}^N$ consisting of eigenvectors of $A^T A$.*

Proof. For (i), suppose the vector $\mathbf{v} \neq \mathbf{0}$ in $\mathbb{R}^N$ satisfies $A^T A \mathbf{v} = \mu \mathbf{v}$ for some number μ. Since all coordinates of both $\mathbf{v}$ and $A^T A \mathbf{v}$ are real numbers, so μ must also be a real number. Also,

$$\begin{aligned}
\mu \, ||\mathbf{v}||^2 &= \mu \, (\mathbf{v} \bullet \mathbf{v}) = (\mu \mathbf{v}) \bullet \mathbf{v} \\
&= (A^T A \mathbf{v}) \bullet \mathbf{v} = (A\mathbf{v}) \bullet (A\mathbf{v}) \\
&= ||A\mathbf{v}||^2 \geq 0.
\end{aligned}$$

Since $\mathbf{v} \neq \mathbf{0}$, it follows that $\mu = ||A\mathbf{v}||^2 / ||\mathbf{v}||^2 \geq 0$.

For (ii), suppose the (non-negative) numbers $\mu_1 \neq \mu_2$ and the nonzero vectors $\mathbf{v}_1$ and $\mathbf{v}_2$ satisfy $A^T A \mathbf{v}_1 = \mu_1 \mathbf{v}_1$ and $A^T A \mathbf{v}_2 = \mu_2 \mathbf{v}_2$. At least one of μ_1 and μ_2 is nonzero, so, for convenience, suppose $\mu_1 \neq 0$. Then

$$\begin{aligned}
\mathbf{v}_1 \bullet \mathbf{v}_2 &= (1/\mu_1)(\mu_1 \mathbf{v}_1) \bullet \mathbf{v}_2 \\
&= (1/\mu_1)(A^T A \mathbf{v}_1) \bullet \mathbf{v}_2 \\
&= (1/\mu_1)\mathbf{v}_1 \bullet (A^T A \mathbf{v}_2) \text{ (using Theorem B.7)} \\
&= (1/\mu_1)\mathbf{v}_1 \bullet (\mu_2 \mathbf{v}_2) \\
&= (\mu_2/\mu_1)\mathbf{v}_1 \bullet \mathbf{v}_2.
\end{aligned}$$

But $(\mu_2/\mu_1) \neq 1$, so we must have $\mathbf{v}_1 \bullet \mathbf{v}_2 = 0$; that is, $\mathbf{v}_1$ and $\mathbf{v}_2$ are orthogonal.

For (iii), we construct an orthonormal basis for the subspace of eigenvectors corresponding to each eigenvalue of $A^T A$. By (ii), these subspaces are mutually orthogonal, so collectively we now have an orthonormal basis for all of $\mathbb{R}^N$, as desired. (Some crucial details, including the fact that $A^T A$ even *has* an eigenvalue to begin with, have been left out. The interested reader should consult a text on linear algebra, such as [1].) $\square$

Theorem B.10 gives us a particularly nice way to factor the matrix $A^T A$. Specifically, record the (non-negative) eigenvalues of $A^T A$ in decreasing order $\mu_1 \geq \mu_2 \geq \ldots \mu_n \geq 0$, each repeated as many times as the dimension of the corresponding subspace of eigenvectors, on the diagonal of an $N \times N$ matrix D; the remaining entries of D are all 0s. Then let V be an $N \times N$ matrix whose columns $\mathbf{v}_1, \ldots, \mathbf{v}_N$ form an orthonormal basis of $\mathbb{R}^N$ and satisfy $A^T A \mathbf{v}_j = \mu_j \mathbf{v}_j$ for all $j = 1, \ldots, N$, as guaranteed by (iii) in the theorem. In this case, V is invertible, with $V^{-1} = V^T$, and

$$A^T A = VDV^T. \tag{B.4}$$

This is called the *eigenvalue decomposition* of $A^T A$ and is also referred to as *diagonalizing* $A^T A$. Note that $A^T A$ is invertible if, and only if, 0 is not an eigenvalue of $A^T A$, which is equivalent to the matrix D being invertible.

Example B.11. As in Example 9.12, let $A = \begin{bmatrix} 1 & 1 & 0 \\ 1 & 1 & 0 \\ 1 & 0 & 1 \\ 1 & 0 & 1 \end{bmatrix}$. So $A^T A = \begin{bmatrix} 4 & 2 & 2 \\ 2 & 2 & 0 \\ 2 & 0 & 2 \end{bmatrix}$, which

has eigenvalues of 6, 2, and 0. We store these, in decreasing order, in the columns of the diagonal matrix $D = \begin{bmatrix} 6 & 0 & 0 \\ 0 & 2 & 0 \\ 0 & 0 & 0 \end{bmatrix}$. Next we compute corresponding unit-length eigenvectors

and store them as the columns of the matrix $V = \begin{bmatrix} 2/\sqrt{6} & 0 & -1/\sqrt{3} \\ 1/\sqrt{6} & -1/\sqrt{2} & 1/\sqrt{3} \\ 1/\sqrt{6} & 1/\sqrt{2} & 1/\sqrt{3} \end{bmatrix}$. The eigenvalue

decomposition is now given by $A^T A = VDV^{-1}$. Note that V is invertible, with $V^{-1} = V^T$.

B.3 Singular value decomposition

For each eigenvalue μ_j of $A^T A$, with unit eigenvector $\mathbf{v}_j$, we have

$$\|A\mathbf{v}_j\| = \sqrt{A\mathbf{v}_j \bullet A\mathbf{v}_j} = \sqrt{A^T A\mathbf{v}_j \bullet \mathbf{v}_j} = \sqrt{(\mu_j \mathbf{v}_j) \bullet \mathbf{v}_j} = \sqrt{\mu_j},$$

since $\mathbf{v}_j$ is a unit vector. Therefore, for each $j = 1, \ldots, N$, there is a unit vector $\mathbf{u}_j$ such that $A\mathbf{v}_j = \sqrt{\mu_j}\, \mathbf{u}_j$. Moreover, provided that μ_j and μ_k are nonzero, then the corresponding vectors $\mathbf{u}_j$ and $\mathbf{u}_k$ are orthogonal to each other. (This includes the case where $j \neq k$ but $\mu_j = \mu_k$.) Indeed, we compute

$$\mathbf{u}_j \bullet \mathbf{u}_k = \frac{1}{\sqrt{\mu_j \cdot \mu_k}} A\mathbf{v}_j \bullet A\mathbf{v}_k = \frac{1}{\sqrt{\mu_j \cdot \mu_k}} A^T A\mathbf{v}_j \bullet \mathbf{v}_k$$

$$= \frac{1}{\sqrt{\mu_j \cdot \mu_k}} (\mu_j \mathbf{v}_j) \bullet \mathbf{v}_k = \sqrt{\frac{\mu_j}{\mu_k}} (\mathbf{v}_j \bullet \mathbf{v}_k) = 0 ,$$

from the construction of the matrix V. In this way, we construct an $M \times M$ matrix U whose columns, $\mathbf{u}_1, \ldots, \mathbf{u}_M$, form an orthonormal basis for $\mathbb{R}^M$ and satisfy $A\mathbf{v}_j = \sqrt{\mu_j}\,\mathbf{u}_j$ whenever $\mu_j \neq 0$. (The columns of U corresponding to the eigenvalue 0 can actually be any unit vectors that will produce a full orthonormal basis of $\mathbb{R}^M$.) As with V, the matrix U is invertible and $U^{-1} = U^T$.

We need one more ingredient to complete this recipe. For each eigenvalue μ_j of $A^T A$, let $\sigma_j = \sqrt{\mu_j}$ and define an $M \times N$ matrix Σ to have diagonal entries $\sigma_1 \geq \sigma_2 \geq \cdots \geq \sigma_N$ and all remaining entries equal to 0. (By the diagonal entries of Σ, we mean those whose column and row addresses are the same; so $[\Sigma]_{jj} = \sigma_j$. In general, Σ need not be a square matrix.) The numbers $\sigma_j = \sqrt{\mu_j}$ are called the *singular values* of the matrix A. (Again, the singular values of A are the square roots of the eigenvalues of the symmetric matrix $A^T A$.) Putting this all together, we see that $AV = U\Sigma$, or, equivalently,

$$A = U\Sigma V^T. \tag{B.5}$$

This is called the *singular value decomposition*, or SVD, of the matrix A. Another way to express the singular value decomposition of A is as the sum

$$A = \sum_{j=1}^{N} \sigma_j \mathbf{u}_j \mathbf{v}_j^T . \tag{B.6}$$

In this sum, each term $\mathbf{u}_j \mathbf{v}_j^T$ is an $M \times N$ matrix, the product of an $M \times 1$ column vector with a $1 \times N$ row vector. Of course, if $\sigma_j = 0$, then the corresponding summand does not contribute anything. So, if $\sigma_1 \geq \ldots \geq \sigma_r > 0$ are the nonzero singular values (and $\sigma_{r+1} = \ldots = \sigma_N = 0$), then we have

$$A = \sum_{j=1}^{r} \sigma_j \mathbf{u}_j \mathbf{v}_j^T . \tag{B.7}$$

This form of the singular value decomposition is also known as the *outer product expansion* of A.

Remark B.12. The singular value decomposition has a geometric interpretation that stems from thinking of the $M \times N$ matrix A as a linear transformation mapping $\mathbb{R}^N$ into $\mathbb{R}^M$. In this view, A maps the N-dimensional unit sphere of $\mathbb{R}^N$ (the set $\{\mathbf{x} \in \mathbb{R}^N : ||\mathbf{x}|| = 1\}$) onto an r-dimensional ellipsoid sitting inside $\mathbb{R}^M$, where r is the number of nonzero singular values of A. The principal axes of this ellipsoid lie in the directions of the first r column vectors of the matrix U and have lengths $2 \cdot \sigma_j$, for $j = 1, \ldots, r$. The nullspace of A has dimension $N - r$. The first r columns of V are the unit vectors that A maps to these principal axes. (This is expressed by the relation $A\mathbf{v}_j = \sigma_j\mathbf{u}_j$.) Thus, when we use the columns of V as our (orthogonal) coordinate framework in $\mathbb{R}^N$, and the columns of U as our framework in $\mathbb{R}^M$, then the action of A is described by the simple matrix Σ. One consequence of this is that the largest singular value, σ_1, is equal to the matrix norm of A as a linear transformation. That is, σ_1 is the maximum factor by which the mapping A re-scales the length of any nonzero vector; $\sigma_1 = ||A|| = \max\{||A\mathbf{x}||/||\mathbf{x}|| : \mathbf{x} \neq \mathbf{0}\}$.

Appendix C

Topics for further study

- For a wealth of information about the Radon transform and its generalizations, as well as extensive lists of references on this topic, see the monograph [24] and the book [15]. Investigate the interaction between the Radon transform and the derivative in order to better understand Radon's original inversion formula.
- The Fourier transform, like Fourier series, was developed originally in the study of differential equations related to the propagation and diffusion of heat. The interaction between the Fourier transform and derivatives was mentioned in the exercises but did not figure into the discussion of CT scans. Moreover, the Fourier transform is a primary tool of physicists, astronomers, and engineers that is used to tackle a broad range of problems. See Bracewell's definitive treatise [7], as well as the entertaining book [9], for much more on this topic.
- We have focused on the filtered back-projection algorithm as well as some basic ART techniques. We have not discussed direct Fourier inversion, which takes the central slice theorem (Theorem 6.1) as its starting point. The filtered back projection (Theorem 6.2) is primarily what is used in current practice. Nonetheless, direct Fourier inversion is a worthwhile subject. The article [35] is a good place to start.
- Study the effect of incorporating finite (nonzero) X-ray beam width into the algorithms for CT.
- Investigate the *fan beam*, *spiral beam*, and *cone beam* geometries and their use in CT scan technology. The latter two methods can reduce the radiation exposure time of the patient by collecting data in all three dimensions at once. The books [12] and [32] are good places to start.
- Investigate the use of wavelets, rather than the Fourier transform, in signal analysis. Wavelets are particularly useful for analyzing signals that are of short duration or that come in bursts. Wavelets are also at the core of the signal compression methods used, for example, in the creation of mp3 music and sound files.

© Springer International Publishing Switzerland 2015
T.G. Feeman, *The Mathematics of Medical Imaging*, Springer Undergraduate
Texts in Mathematics and Technology, DOI 10.1007/978-3-319-22665-1

- Study the evolution of the scanning machines themselves, from the earliest EMI scanner designed by Hounsfield to the 5th generation machines that employ electron beam CT. Also, it would be interesting to look more closely at the computational process that is encoded into the scanning machines used in clinical practice.

- In positron emission tomography (PET) and single-photon emission computed tomography (SPECT), a radioactive isotope is introduced internally into the patient. This isotope tends to bind to areas where certain pathologies are present or certain physiological functions are in effect. Positrons are emitted from the sample in pairs moving in opposite directions. When the intensities of a matching pair are measured by external detectors, the sum of the measurements yields a value of the Radon transform along the line defined by the paths of the two particles. Then a modified version of the CT analysis discussed here can be applied to form an image. So PET and SPECT are like inside-out versions of CT. See [30] and [32] for an introduction to these types of tomography.

- The study of Fourier series predates the development of the Fourier transform historically. Though we have alluded to the theory of Fourier series in only a few places in the present work, it nonetheless inspires and informs the transform theory and is a cornerstone of the branch of mathematics known as functional analysis. See [31] and [47] to get started.

- Functional MRI (fMRI) exploits the difference in the magnetic response of nuclei contained in oxygenated blood compared to those in deoxygenated blood. Increased neuronal activity requires a rapid influx of oxygen to the area of the activity, where the additional oxygen is consumed by the active neurons. MRI images that portray these magnetic variations are created during many repetitions of some activity or experience, such as performing mental arithmetic. Then statistical methods are used to determine which areas of the brain can reliably be said to be most active during the activity.

- For the strongest versions of many of the theorems in Chapters 5 and 7, as well as for a careful error analysis of the discrete approximations discussed in Chapter 8, we would require a deeper understanding of the spaces L^1 and L^2 of integrable functions and of the theory of integral operators and kernel functions. The books [2] and [46] can help get one pointed in the right direction.

- Use R to develop additional implementations of the image reconstruction algorithms studied in this book. We make no claim that the code used here is the most efficient possible. Also, nothing has been said about incorporating the matrix forms and the fast Fourier transform, discussed in Chapter 8, into the implementations. One might also explore how to manage data collected via the fan beam or other geometry. Generating computer images for magnetic resonance imaging is another avenue for exploration.

Bibliography

1. Axler, S.: Linear Algebra Done Right, 3rd edn. Springer, New York (2015)
2. Bartle, R.G.: The Elements of Real Analysis, 2nd edn. Wiley, New York (1976)
3. Bauschke, H.H., Borwein, J.M.: On projection algorithms for solving convex feasibility problems. SIAM Rev. **38**, 367–426 (1996)
4. Bloch, F., Hansen, W.W., Packard, M.: Nuclear induction. Phys. Rev. **69**, 127 (1946)
5. Blümich, B.: NMR Imaging of Materials. Oxford University Press, Oxford (2000)
6. Bracewell, R.N.: Image reconstruction in radio astronomy. In: Herman, G.T. (ed.) Image Reconstruction from Projections: Implementation and Applications. Topics in Applied Physics, vol. 32. Springer, Berlin (1979)
7. Bracewell, R.N.: The Fourier Transform and Its Applications, 3rd edn. McGraw-Hill, Boston (2000)
8. Bracewell, R.N., Riddle, A.C.: Inversion of fan-beam scans in radio astronomy. Astrophys. J. **150**, 427–434 (1967)
9. Butz, T.: Fourier Transformation for Pedestrians. Springer, Berlin (2006)
10. Censor, Y.: Row-action methods for huge and sparse systems and their applications. SIAM Rev. **23**, 444–464 (1981)
11. Censor, Y.: Finite series-expansion reconstruction methods. Proc. IEEE **71**, 409–419 (1983)
12. Cierniak, R.: X-Ray Computed Tomography in Biomedical Engineering. Springer, New York (2011)
13. Cooley, T.W., Tukey, J.W.: An algorithm for the machine calculation of complex Fourier series. Math. Comput. **19**, 297–301 (1965)
14. Cormack, A.M.: Representation of a function by its line integrals, with some radiological applications I, II. J. Appl. Phys. **34**, 2722–2727 (1963); **35**, 2908–2912 (1964)
15. Deans, S.R.: The Radon Transform and Some of Its Applications. Krieger, Malabar (1993); reprinted by Dover, Mineola (2007)
16. Dewdney, A.K.: How to resurrect a cat from its grin, in Mathematical Recreations. Sci. Am. **263**(3), 174–177 (1990). Note: In the first edition, I incorrectly ascribed this to Martin Gardner. My thanks go to Y. Le Du, from France, for being a devoted Martin Gardner fan and pointing out to me that Gardner was no longer writing his Mathematical Games column for Scientific American in 1990
17. Epstein, C.L.: Introduction to the Mathematics of Medical Imaging, 2nd edn. SIAM, Philadelphia (2008)
18. Feeman, T.G.: Conformality, the exponential function, and world map projections. Coll. Math. J. **32**, 334–342 (2001)
19. Feeman, T.G.: On a family of circles. Primus **21**, 193–196 (2011)
20. Freeman, R.: Magnetic Resonance in Chemistry and Medicine. Oxford University Press, Oxford (2003)
21. Gadian, D.G.: Nuclear Magnetic Resonance and Its Applications to Living Systems. Oxford University Press, Oxford (1982)

© Springer International Publishing Switzerland 2015
T.G. Feeman, *The Mathematics of Medical Imaging*, Springer Undergraduate
Texts in Mathematics and Technology, DOI 10.1007/978-3-319-22665-1

22. Gordon, R., Bender, R., Herman, G.T.: Algebraic reconstruction techniques (ART) for three-dimensional electron microscopy and X-ray photography. J. Theor. Biol. **29**, 471–481 (1970)
23. Hansen, P.C., Nagy, J.G., O'Leary, D.P.: Deblurring Images: Matrices, Spectra, and Filtering. SIAM, Philadelphia (2006)
24. Helgason, S.: The Radon Transform, 2nd edn. Birkhäuser, Boston (1999)
25. Herman, G.T., Lent, A., Rowland, S.W.: ART: mathematics and applications. J. Theor. Biol. **42**, 1–32 (1973)
26. Hinshaw, W.S., Lent, A.H.: An introduction to NMR imaging: from the Bloch equation to the imaging equation. Proc. IEEE **71**, 338–350 (1983)
27. Hounsfield, G.N.: Computerized transverse axial scanning tomography. Br. J. Radiol. **46**, 1016–1022 (1973)
28. Hounsfield, G.N.: A method of and apparatus for examination of a body by radiation such as X or gamma radiation. The Patent Office, London (1972). Patent Specification 1283915
29. Kalman, D.: A singularly valuable decomposition: the SVD of a matrix. Coll. Math. J. **27**, 2–23 (1996)
30. Knoll, G.F.: Single-photon emission computed tomography. Proc. IEEE **71**, 320–329 (1983)
31. Körner, T.W.: Fourier Analysis. Cambridge University Press, Cambridge (1988)
32. Kuchment, P.: The Radon Transform and Medical Imaging. CBMS, vol. 85. SIAM, Philadelphia (2014)
33. Kuperman, V.: Magnetic Resonance Imaging: Physical Principles and Applications. Academic Press, San Diego (2000)
34. Lauterbur, P.C.: Image formation by induced local interactions: examples employing nuclear magnetic resonance. Nature **242**, 190 (1973)
35. Lewitt, R.M.: Reconstruction algorithms: transform methods. Proc. IEEE **71**, 390–408 (1983)
36. Louis, A.K.: Nonuniqueness in inverse Radon problems: the frequency distribution of the ghosts. Math. Z. **185**, 429–440 (1984)
37. Louis, A.K.: Approximate inverse for linear and some nonlinear problems. Inverse Prob. **12**, 175–190 (1996)
38. Mansfield, P.: Multi-planar image formation using NMR spin echoes. J. Phys. C. **10**, L55 (1977)
39. Natterer, F.: The Mathematics of Computerized Tomography. Classics in Applied Mathematics, vol. 32. SIAM, Philadelphia (2001)
40. Noble, B., Daniel, J.W.: Applied Linear Algebra, 3rd edn. Prentice-Hall, Englewood Cliffs (1988)
41. Purcell, E.M., Torrey, H.C., Pound, R.V.: Resonance absorption by nuclear magnetic moments in a solid. Phys. Rev. **69**, 37 (1946)
42. R Core Team, R: A Language and Environment for Statistical Computing. R Foundation for Statistical Computing, Vienna (2014). http://www.R-project.org
43. Radon, J.: Über die Bestimmung von Funktionen durch ihre Integralwerte längs gewisserMannigfaltigkeiten. Berichte Sächsische Akademie der Wissenschaften **69**, 262–277 (1917)
44. Ramachandran, G.N., Lakshminarayanan, A.V.: Three-dimensional reconstruction from radiographs and electron micrographs II: application of convolutions instead of Fourier transforms. Proc. Natl. Acad. Sci. USA **68**, 2236–2240 (1971)
45. Rowland, S.W.: Computer implementation of image reconstruction formulas. In: Herman, G.T. (ed.) Image Reconstruction from Projections: Implementation and Applications. Topics in Applied Physics, vol. 32. Springer, Berlin (1979)
46. Rudin, W.: Real and Complex Analysis, 2nd edn. McGraw-Hill, New York (1974)
47. Seeley, R.: An Introduction to Fourier Series and Integrals. W.A. Benjamin, New York (1966)
48. Shepp, L.A., Kruskal, J.B.: Computerized tomography: the new medical X-ray technology. Am. Math. Mon. **34**, 35–44 (1978)
49. Shepp, L.A., Logan, B.F.: The Fourier reconstruction of a head section. IEEE Trans. Nucl. Sci. **NS-21**, 21–43 (1974)
50. Strang, G.: The Fundamental Theorem of Linear Algebra. Am. Math. Mon. **100**, 848–855 (1993)
51. Trefethen, L.N., Bau, D. III: Numerical Linear Algebra. SIAM, Philadelphia (1997)
52. Wang, L.: Cross-section reconstruction with a fan-beam scanning geometry. IEEE Trans. Comput. **C-26**, 264–268 (1977)

Index

© Springer International Publishing Switzerland 2015
T.G. Feeman, *The Mathematics of Medical Imaging*, Springer Undergraduate
Texts in Mathematics and Technology, DOI 10.1007/978-3-319-22665-1

Printed in the United States
By Bookmasters